Choosing
NOT
Cheating

The Beverly Hills Eat for Pleasure

Slim for Life Plan

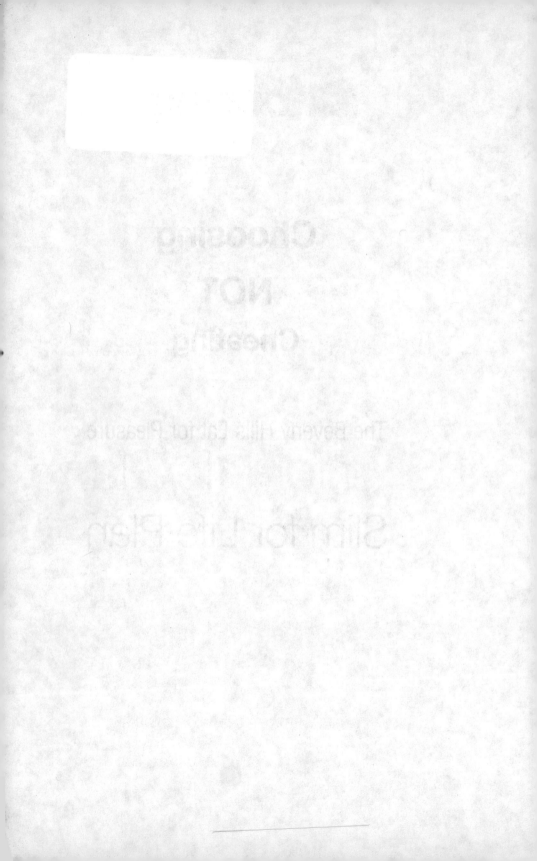

Choosing
NOT
Cheating

The Beverly Hills Eat for Pleasure

Slim for Life Plan

by Midge Elias

HUMANICS LIMITED   ATLANTA GEORGIA

Humanics New Age is an imprint of Humanics Limited

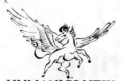

HUMANICS NEW AGE
P.O. BOX 7447
Atlanta, Georgia 30309

First Edition

PRINTED IN THE UNITED STATES OF AMERICA

Library of Congress Cataloging-in-Publication Data

Elias, Midge, -(date.)
    Choosing not cheating : the Beverly Hills eat for pleasure,
slim for life plan / by Midge Elias.

    p.   cm.
Bibliography: p.
1. Reducing diets—Recipes.   I. Title.
RM222.2.E43   1989   641.5′635—dc20   89-15462CIP
ISBN 0-89334-130-4

Cover Photo by Ranjit Ahuja

Dedication

To my clients
Who give my life new meaning
When their lives change

Table of Contents

Foreword

In *Choosing Not Cheating*, Midge Elias gives us an effective diet and exercise plan for a thinner and healthier life. She is able to describe in a clear and understandable manner, a nutrition plan that is both medically sound and practically effective.

Clinically, most physicians are urging their patients to adopt diets lower in fat and protein and higher in complex carbohydrates and fiber. (This is particularly true for most patients with obesity, diabetes, cardiac and kidney diseases.)

Why are these diets important to our patients? Consider the scientific evidence. Fat, whether animal or vegetable in origin, is calorie-dense, containing nearly two and one-half times the calories as the same weight of carbohydrate. And, although protein has the same calorie-to-weight ratio as carbohydrate, most dietary protein is either surrounded by or marbled with fat. Besides, most Americans eat far more protein than their bodies (or kidneys) need. High-fiber foods (those recommended in this book) tend to improve glucose tolerance, to lower cholesterol, and to decrease the risk of certain bowel disorders.

Most physicians also strongly urge aerobic exercise programs tailored to each patient's age and medical status. Appropriate exercise improves weight control, strengthens muscles, helps physical endurance, prevents bone loss, and adds to the overall well-being.

In *Choosing Not Cheating*, Midge explains how to practically adopt these sound nutritional and exercise ideas to a life-style that works in America today. There is no need to totally give up special treats or calorie-inefficient recipes. Rather, one rations them to special occasions roughly 20% of our diet—whenever we decide that a particular food is special enough to be worth the extra calories it may "cost."

We are taught to opt for filling, nutritious, satisfying foods as a way of life. We are given clues and cues on how to eat in or eat out, how to fill up but not fill out. We learn why certain foods and nutrients are more valuable than others. We learn how certain food preparations are more calorically "expensive" than others. We are given examples of life situations and nutritional solutions as they actually affected patients in Midge's practice.

For the past few years, Midge has been a nutritionist-consultant to many of my diabetic and metabolic patients. I watched her apply the principles she describes in this book, and have counted up a considerable success rate—success with prolonged weight loss, long-term metabolic control, exercise enhancement, and overall life-style improvement.

As our patients begin their nutrition programs, we refer to them as actively "Midgeing." People start out to achieve a certain weight goal, but they continue because they like being in control of their weight, their exercise, and their bodies. You, too, can share these positive feelings. So good luck, good metabolism, and good "Midgeing."

Arthur N. Lurvey

Arthur N. Lurvey, M.D.

Arthur Lurvey, M.D., is in private practice in Beverly Hills. He is a Diplomate of the American Board of Internal Medicine, the American Board of Endocrinology and Metabolism, and former Chief-of-Staff of Midway Hospital in Los Angeles. Dr. Lurvey personally adopted the Choosing Not Cheating lifestyle two years ago, has sustained a weight loss of approximately thirty pounds, and a drop in cholesterol of 30%.

Acknowledgements

My thanks to the following people:

Julie Prendiville, my catalyst, for providing the spark that ignited this project

Meredith Loring, a talented editor, who nurtured both me and my manuscript.

Peter Kraus, M.D., for confidence in me very early in my career.

Susan and Arthur Lurvey, M.D., a brilliant medical team of extraordinary compassion and humanity.

My husband, Allan, children: Eric, Dan and Bettina, my parents, Edith and Lewis Rowen and Sara and Eli Elias for their love and support while I pursued this very personal odyssey.

Susan Letton Upchurch, the apotheosis of friendship.

A Faerie Tale

For Dieters

Once upon a time, a young prince went forth to seek his fortune. After many years of searching, he saw on the horizon a beautiful shining city. As he drew nearer, there appeared a golden palace set on a lush green hillside where beautiful maidens frolicked on the grass. Bluebirds and rainbows could be seen overhead.

Knowing somehow that this place was where he must be, he rushed headlong down the only road leading to the city. Suddenly a powerful dragon appeared, blocking his way. But no obstacle was too formidable for the prince. He drew his sword, and with a mighty stroke, slew the dragon, continuing triumphantly into the city of many pleasures. Naturally, he lived happily ever after. Because this is a faerie tale.

You are a seeker on that road. You can see the magic city where people seem to lead enchanted lives. They eat delicious food, go out to restaurants and enjoy parties and holidays. They have lots of energy, look great in tight jeans, and never go on a diet. You want so much to be a part of that place that has for so long eluded you.

1

But you, too, have a dragon to slay. Your dragon is your reluctance to change. If you've been doing things in a certain way for a long time, it is wrenchingly difficult to force yourself to act differently.

You might have thought that exercise was for other people, and that you could be slim through dieting alone.

You might have thought that pills or drinking strange concoctions was the way to suppress an unwelcome appetite.

You might have felt that you were doomed to being fat because of your piggish overeating or bad heredity.

Now you are going to learn something different. All you must do is conquer your resistance to making changes. Trust what you will read in the following pages until you can rely on yourself. Eat the right foods, and exercise even though it might feel uncomfortable in the beginning.

Soon, positive results will convince you that at last you have entered the magic city. You can do it! **You** can conquer the problem of overweight forever. This happy ending is within your power to achieve.

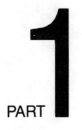

PART **1** the **Basics**

1

The Beverly Hills

State of Mind

Eat Everything and Be Slim

Oh no, not another diet book from Beverly Hills. Hasn't this been done?

Is the geographical origin of an eating plan really relevant?

In this case it is. And this is not a diet book. It's a program that has enabled some very glamorous people—all kinds of people—to deal successfully with food.

In many ways, Beverly Hills *is* the magic place portrayed in the media. Magnificent homes, exclusive boutiques, and more of the world's expensive cars than anywhere else on earth can be found in this sun-washed, glittering corner of the world. It is the "hometown" of some very beautiful, very rich, highly visible people, going about their professional and private lives. Not only performers, but those who work around them—agents, writers, producers, and attorneys—are intensely concerned about "image." They have to look good in their expensive (if casual) clothes, but being thin isn't enough; they want to look sleek and healthy and forever young. After all, it was here in Hollywood that the dream of the golden girl and her handsome, sun-bronzed prince was born; it is from here that these images become models for the rest of the country and the world.

But here in Beverly Hills, there is an opposing force at work: the emphasis on and the abundance of DELICIOUS FOOD. As a major food capital of the nation, California is an incubator of the newest culinary trends. The restaurant scene is very important in the entertainment business—deal-making breakfasts, power lunches, and evenings spent at the trendiest spots. Innovative chefs oblige by offering an endless array of temptations, and Beverly Hills people participate in the festivities to the fullest. Most restaurateurs agree that people in this area order desserts after dinner with greater frequency than anywhere else in the country.

In addition, there are fantastic food markets displaying almost anything one could want to eat, including probably the world's finest produce; counters where you can indulge your fancy for luscious cakes and pastries, fresh-baked breads, exotic cheeses, and fancy chocolate.

And yet, people in the public eye feel they must look lean in their designer jeans as they push the shopping cart around the store. They must be glamourous and slim as they make their entrance into a restaurant. How can they participate in this "food fiesta" and still be fit? Why are some people lucky enough to accomplish this, while you may be struggling endlessly with your weight, always dieting so you can't have any fun, or bingeing and feeling fat? Have Beverly Hills people discovered a way to enjoy food and still be slim? I wrote this book because I want you to share the Beverly Hills state of mind that says,

YOU CAN HAVE IT ALL!

I am a practicing behavioral counselor and nutrition consultant in Beverly Hills, specializing in weight control. Since being slim is an absolute necessity for many of the people I work with, they have tried just about everything to reach their goal. However, I have seen the disappointing results and the emotional pain produced by almost every popular diet plan and know there is a tremendous need for a new approach. Perhaps you, too, have been on the diet merry-go-round but have never succeeded in permanently controlling your weight.

Although the diets vary in content and format, they have one thing in common. They elicit feelings of dread. You know you must once again bite the bullet of self-denial, suspending all fun until that magic moment when you are slim. Sadly, that moment (so painfully if ever achieved) is usually fleeting. The "diet" is over, so your old eating habits return, quickly reshaping your new body back to the old. The discouraging data show that 95% of people who lose weight do not succeed in maintaining that loss. Why? There are two equally important reasons: new eating patterns are never learned, and human needs are not adequately met.

The Choosing Not Cheating Plan is unique and effective because it deals with people **the way they really are.** It is in conflict with neither the powerful force of raw animal hunger, nor the psychological needs of human nature. It offers no short-term crutches such as pills, powders, or packaged foods. This Plan is designed to help you only until you are ready to handle the abundant, tempting food world on your own with confidence instead of dread.

People everywhere are better informed about nutrition and the proper care of their bodies than they were in the past. Perhaps the time for fads and quick weight-loss plans is over. After following enough convoluted schemes, and never winning the endless struggle, (Have you gained and lost the same ten pounds for years?) you are probably ready to try something different; something that works.

The Facts About Eating

- The primary purpose of food is to nourish the body.
- Dining can be raised to an art and a delight for the senses.
- Eating is meant to be fun.
- Sometimes people eat for emotional reasons.
- Most people want to be slim.

Can these seemingly conflicting needs be reconciled? Can eating serve all these masters? The answer is a very definite YES. Slimness and optimum health can coexist with the pressures of our times and the pleasures of living the good life. You CAN have a new, positive relationship with food, free of deprivation, "will power," and guilt.

I believe that everybody can be slim, and that people have a right to enjoy food as an important pleasurable part of life. I have helped many people here in Beverly Hills "have it all," and conquer their weight problem forever. Let me help you too.

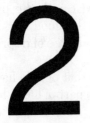

Choosing Not Cheating

The Plan

Principles

Here are the principles upon which the Choosing Not Cheating Plan is built:

1. Never go on a diet.
Anything you have to go "on" is something you eventually will have to go "off." To lose weight and permanently maintain that loss, you must adopt a livable lifetime plan that allows you to be a **social animal** as well as a **healthy** one.

2. Make exercise an integral part of your life.
An appropriate form of aerobic exercise, executed properly four to seven times a week, is essential to weight loss, weight maintenance, and the highest levels of physical and mental health.

3. While food is a source of great pleasure, it is primarily for nourishment.
Without the proper nutrients, vibrant health cannot be maintained. Apparently, our bodies have changed very little since

primitive times, but the foods we eat have changed drastically. We overconsume fats, sugar, salt, and processed foods, but humankind in his natural state ate primarily a diet of grains, vegetables, and fruits supplemented from time to time with fish and meat. For optimum health and ideal weight, most of what we eat should once again be these health-giving complex carbohydrates, eaten as whole foods in their natural, unprocessed and unadulterated state whenever possible.

4.   Rely on your body's own internal cues.

Learn when you are physiologically (not emotionally) hungry, what your body really wants to eat, and when you are comfortably full. I will show you how.

5.   Adopt the 80/20% way of life.

Allow yourself festive times within the framework of your healthy eating style. If 80% of your diet consists of fresh, health-giving foods, 20% of your calories can be spent indulging in life's "party" situations. These percentages are flexible, and should be modified to suit individual needs, situations, and times.

6.   Never waste calories.

You are the best, so don't spend your calories on foods of lesser value. Since calories **are** spent on everything you eat, your guideline should be: *Is this really worth it?* Whether it is a healthful, low-calorie choice or a festive high-calorie one, make sure that the quality is exactly what you deserve. A peach should be the most perfect one you can find; a piece of chocolate should be exactly the kind you crave.

7.   Study people who are naturally slim.

Who better to tell you how to be a slim, fit person than one who is just that? If you wanted to make money, you'd ask the advice of a self-made millionaire. Don't spend your time commiserating with other overweight people about your mutual plight. Instead, adopt patterns that slim people have successfully integrated into their lives, and then take **ACTION**.

All Needs Considered

The evidence is in and it's overwhelming. A diet high in complex carbohydrates, very low in fats, and without any refined sugar or artificial ingredients, is the ideal one for human beings to follow.

And yet it is also a fact that people have a strong need for pleasure and fun. All over the world, special times revolve around food. At every ceremony, every holiday, every special day, the celebration of food is the celebration of life.

To try to live the no-fat, no-sugar, no-chemicals way 100% of the time is a fine idea, but in reality, it's almost impossible to do. Human nature says "If you deprive me, I will rebel; if you restrict me for too long, I will throw away your plan."

Life is to be enjoyed. Part of that enjoyment comes from having a slim, healthy body you can be proud of. Another part comes from the freedom to stroll down the street on a sunny summer afternoon enjoying an ice cream cone, feeling pleasure, not guilt.

Recognizing the realities of human nature, and the fact that we live in the modern world, our job is to formulate a way of eating that considers **all** your needs as you go through life—the need to have a body that is slim and fit, and the need to enjoy special dinners, parties, weddings, and just plain eating for fun. Eating for pleasure and being slim must comfortably coexist, or no "diet" will ever succeed.

Changing Your Life: The CNC Plan

On this Plan, approximately 80% of the time you will be eating foods that provide maximum nutrition for the lowest number of calories—mostly complex carbohydrates. Since these grains, vegetables, legumes, and fruits are the foods that contain fiber, you will feel full and satisfied, never hungry. Instead of being the centerpiece of the meal, lean meats are used sparingly, and fats of all kind are kept to a minimum. Dietary experts are in agreement that this style of eating promotes the highest level of health, and the maintenance of body weight.

Since our bodies were designed to eat natural foods, after a few weeks you will be very happy eating in this manner. Your delicious mango, or warm, welcoming bowl of lentil soup will be appreciated as much in its own way as any festive restaurant meal.

Whatever constitutes your idea of treats and special tastes, you are encouraged to enjoy them for roughly 20% of the food you consume. These percentages are variable, depending on how quickly you want to lose weight, and what is going on in your life at the time.

My belief is that neither style of eating should stand alone—a diet where either mode eclipses the other is out of balance. Carrots will never replace chocolate, and each has a place in a fit, healthy life. But too much chocolate and not enough vegetables leads to obesity and a reduced level of health.

Since the "20%" kinds of food are likely to be high in fat and calories, they had better bring you maximum pleasure. It helps you to think of calories as money. Of course you want to get the most for what you "buy." When you go out for dinner in a restaurant, it had better be wonderful! When you eat cookies, stale ones won't do. Remember that while the calories remain constant whether stale or fresh, the pleasure does not. Because you have only a limited percentage of your food budget to spend on these "treats," you can't afford to be less than choosy.

Why You Will Succeed This Time

- You don't have to put your life on hold. You can continue to live fully while losing weight.

- You will never go hungry, or have to use will power to keep from eating.

- You are encouraged to eat complex carbohydrates such as potatoes, pasta, rice, whole-grain bread, and beans. These are "soothing," filling foods so you never feel deprived, or as though you are "on a diet."

- You will learn that by exercising, you get to eat more!

What You Really Want to Eat Will Change

You will find that your preferences do undergo changes, without any effort on your part. By spending 80% of your time eating in a healthy, natural style, where fresh, whole foods predominate, former favorites begin to taste too sweet, rich, or greasy. But some will remain special forever. Who would voluntarily choose to live in a world without ice cream, champagne, pizza, or pasta? Or travel to France, and not sample bread, wine or Brie? But you may have no difficulty deciding that fat-laden fast foods, doughnuts, and potato chips are no longer worth their high caloric cost.

You will be eating in a free, less-structured way, more in tune with your body's internal signals. You might decide to have a banana and a baked potato for lunch, or a giant salad and brown rice for dinner.

That is why you **won't** find a rigid diet plan in this book. No one diet can be right for everyone. You **will** find guidelines on nutrition and food selection—the information you need to navigate yourself through a successful weight-loss program. You will no longer need to rely on a weight-loss center, a powdered supplement clinic, or a printed menu to tell you when, how, and what to eat. You will not be forced to write down every bite you consume, weigh and measure each portion, or slavishly compute calories. This plan is not a system of food substitutions that require accounting skills to follow. But, if you want to, you will lose weight—the right way, the lasting way.

I know that your desire to be slim and healthy is not the only need in your life. You interact with other people; you participate in life right now, not later, after some mythical goal weight is achieved. Some days, some meals, some treats will be, by your choice, higher calorie. You will know that these events are simply a normal component of a full life, and that they belong to you, never to be taken away. Once that realization occurs, you will never have to say, "I've been good, I've been bad" or "I cheated." You will finally act like the rational adult that you are, comfortable with food and capable of reaching and maintaining your ideal weight.

3

How to **Choose**

Instead of **Cheat**

Signals From Within

In the wild an animal knows exactly when it is hungry. The signals from an empty stomach propel it to seek its species' proper nourishment. When it has had enough, it stops eating. It's a rather simple mechanism that works very well, so that in their natural state animals suffer neither from eating disorders nor obesity. You only find fat animals in zoos or in people's homes as pets.

We, too, are animals. Human babies cry to be fed, and stop sucking when their stomachs are full. Every parent has observed how infants will spit out their nipples when they have had enough, refusing to suck even one drop more.

Newborns eat because of the same true physiological hunger that motivates all animals. It is only later in life, when eating occurs for *other* reasons, that problems arise. Sometimes our perfect, natural mechanisms of knowing when we are hungry, what it is we want to eat, and when we've had enough, become distorted. This distortion occurs when we eat to please others— eating the foods selections and the amounts that others choose for us, involuntary membership in the clean-plate club, "concern" for starving people throughout the world, inflexible dining hours, pressure to finish one kind of food before "treats" are allowed. Perhaps the most common mistake is teaching a child by words or example that eating will soothe hurt feelings. The simple act of consoling an unhappy child with a cookie is the first step toward pairing food with emotions instead of with its natural stimulus, true physiological hunger.

Life in our culture is terribly complex and, of course, you can't always act like an animal in the wild. You will, at times, eat for "the wrong reasons." But it is still of paramount importance that you reestablish contact with your body's own trustworthy signals. Try to peel back the layers of civilization, find your healthy animal-self underneath, and tune in to the messages your body sends you.

Awareness Questions

Ask yourself these questions to help heighten your awareness:

1.   Am I hungry?
2.   Am I eating on cue?
3.   What do I want?
4.   Do I like it?
5.   Am I full?

Let's look at each of these questions in depth.

1. Am I Hungry

At the moment that I am about to eat, am I feeling true physiological hunger, or is it thirst, boredom, anger, loneliness, fatigue, tension, despair, or joy?

As a baby, you started out with that perfect system: physiological hunger made you eat, fullness made you stop, and your body weight was exactly what it was supposed to be. Then other people started getting in the way, deciding what, when, and how much you should eat. Mom may have believed that the only healthy baby was a fat baby. She might have induced you to eat more than you wanted to by:

Games

"Eat this bite for daddy, this one for grandma."

"Here comes the airplane" (spoon), "zooming into the hangar" (baby's mouth).

"Watch this toy" (to distract you), while food gets shoved in your mouth.

"If you finish everything, you get to be in the clean-plate club." (This was also a favored technique in schools and camps.)

Bribes

"You can't go out to play (or watch television) until after you've finished your dinner."

"If you eat all your vegetables, you can have dessert" (giving rise to the thought that dessert is good, veggies are bad).

Guilt

"Children are starving all over the world, and you won't even finish your dinner."

"In this family, we don't waste food—it costs too much."

"I worked all day and then came home to cook this for you—some thanks I get."

"Look, your brother eats everything; he's a good boy."

For everyone, food and emotions are linked together to some degree, but for some people, emotion has **replaced** hunger as the primary stimulus for eating. It is not really difficult to see how these patterns become established.

When babies are being fed, they are usually held and cuddled and are the total focus of attention. Food and feeding time get paired with feeling good, being soothed, being taken care of. Eating becomes irrevocably associated with comfort. Food equals love.

When a toddler cries, he is diverted with a treat. Children are rewarded for being "good" with a trip to buy ice cream, and for being "bad" with no dessert. A television commercial shows a sad little boy who's had a rough day at school being consoled by his mother with a sweet drink. One catchy little jingle suggests that oven baked foods are the same as love. Another national company suggests that if you are feeling blue, cheer yourself up with a box of their chocolates.

Thus, through powerful early conditioning, the strands of eating and feelings are interwoven. Celebrations and accomplishments are rewarded by festive eating. For some people food can lessen emotional pain and keep tension and fear at bay, at least for a time. People may let you down, but food can always be counted on to keep you company.

It appears as though some people use food to "fill a hole in the soul." And it works. For a moment, the bad feelings are banished, and the baby-comfort returns. But then—so soon— the negative cycle begins. Loneliness, anger, fear and boredom are now accompanied by self-disgust. The greater the quantity eaten, the more "sinful" the food, the stronger the feelings of weakness and failure. And what is the defense against these feelings? More eating, of course.

Maybe someday, like an animal in the wild, you too will eat only in response to physical hunger. Maybe not. In many cases, the "wrong reasons" continue to trigger eating throughout life. But there are positive, successful ways to deal with this issue, so that it won't prevent you from finally controlling your weight.

How to Binge With the Least Damage

Instead of making doomed resolutions to stop being an "emotional" eater, prepare yourself in advance for the next time the dangerous feelings descend—those times when you know that nothing can get between you and food. Make only one decision: to change the choices of the foods you use to "fill the hole." Put carbohydrates to work for you. Most important, *avoid all fats of any kind.*

Decide to eat a whole loaf of bread if necessary, or many plates of pasta without oil or butter. Make an enormous bowl of air-popped popcorn. Try three baked potatoes covered with ketchup, mustard or salsa. Eat any non-sugary carbohydrate— bread, rolls, crackers with pure fruit jam, and have a lot of liquid along with it, like cups of a hot beverage, or large glasses of a cold drink. Just that one modification in behavior—keeping away from fats at these critical times—will cut your caloric consumption way down.

These non-fat foods, eaten in sufficient quantities, will effectively bury the bad feelings. The soothing fullness will be there, but the self-disgust will be absent. When you compute the calories of the "binge", you will be pleasantly surprised. No matter how much bread, potatoes, or popcorn you eat at one time, the calories will not even be in the same ballpark with fast-food hamburgers, fries, pizza, ice cream, and other fatty foods. This single behavior change will begin a positive, upward cycle toward permanent weight control.

The Mighty Hunger Drive

Overweight people have learned not to trust the hunger drive. It has let you down in the past—led to overeating and being fat. You train yourself to block it, ignore it, deny it. Many clients tell me they honestly don't know what actual hunger feels like. The moment they feel any sort of discomfort, they perceive it as hunger, and put something in the mouth as quickly as possible.

Every time you're about to eat, think, "Am I really physically hungry? If I were a carnivorous animal, would I make a kill right now?" If you're not sure, get a drink of water, and ask yourself again in ten minutes. Your job is to get back in tune with your body's messages—to turn up their volume instead of burying them. When you know that you are feeling real physical hunger, eat as soon as possible. Don't allow yourself to get over-hungry. When blood sugar gets low, you may get weak, both physically and mentally, and it is at those times that out-of-control eating happens—anything and everything is consumed, too fast, and without discrimination. Start to take the best care of yourself, and don't allow this to happen.

One day I was a guest lecturer at a weight-reduction center that demanded adherence to a very rigid program. A woman in the audience was having difficulty with the prohibition against any eating after 6:00 P.M. She was a night person, she said, not going to sleep until about 2:00 A.M. Her hunger would increase as the night wore on. When asked my advice, I suggested that she rearrange her eating schedule to conform more realistically with her life. But the company's representative in the audience disagreed, saying that deviation from procedure was not permissible under any circumstances.

"What advice," I asked, "do **YOU** have for the lady who is attempting to go for eight hours without eating?"

"We suggest a warm bath", she answered.

I was relieved when laughter erupted spontaneously among the assembled dieters. Here was an "expert" actually advising the denial of one of the body's most powerful signals. Practically speaking, for how many nights can you drown hunger in a bubble bath?

You know that kind of "will-power" never works. Only when you live in harmony with your body's needs and messages and **stop trying to fight them** will you finally get slim and stay that way forever.

A client named Irene touched me deeply when she confided that every morning she prayed for enough strength not to eat anything that day. How much more on target it would be to pray for the ability to hear the body's signals, and the wisdom to know how to nourish yourself with healthy, low-calorie foods.

2. Am I Eating on Cue?

Am I a prisoner of other people's routines and schedules, sometimes waiting too long for food, sometimes eating just because it's convenient?

• You never want breakfast until 10:00 A.M., but by then you're locked in at work or school.

• You're hungry for dinner at 6:00 P.M. but 8:30 is the fashionable time to dine.

• You're ready for lunch at 11:30 A.M. but your scheduled break is at 1:00 P.M.

• The clock says it's dinner time, and everyone must sit down at the table, hungry or not.

Life is complicated, and it **IS** difficult sometimes to eat when you really want to. But it is vital to follow your natural hunger rhythms whenever you can.

Your Particular Eating Pattern

Do you prefer little snacks all day long to large meals at one sitting? Many slim people eat this way. In fact, it is probably most natural for the human species to continually "graze" in the style of our foraging ancestors. Studies have shown that those who eat one big meal in the evening tend to be overweight and have higher cholesterol levels than those who nibble throughout the day whenever they feel hungry.

Each family member is on a different schedule these days—two careers, school, part-time jobs, sports, social life. The result may be that the whole family assembled at the table for meals is a rarity rather than an everyday occurrence. These times together are special and important, but in fact, "independent eating" is a very viable family pattern. As long as the refrigerator and the pantry are well-stocked, no one has to function as a short-order cook. In this flexible style, each person has an opportunity to decide what and when he or she feels like eating.

It is even easier for single people to tune into their own unique needs and shop, cook, or dine out according to what feels right on that day, at that particular meal.

Of course when children are small, meals must be provided, but mothers report that their children show clear individual preferences very early. Many children go through phases where they want the same foods over and over, or when they seem to want to eat practically nothing. The research has shown that with good nourishing foods available and minimum pressure from concerned parents, children will choose a healthy diet in the long run.

If you were the victim of faulty early training, break the cycle and do better in your own family. What greater gift could you give to your child than a healthy attitude toward food, where eating is never done to please, punish, or soothe emotions; when hunger is the only cue for eating; where food choices are determined by the body's needs, and the meal is over when the body is pleasantly full.

Don't be afraid to make some unorthodox modifications in your schedule to become more responsive to body signals. If you keep your own behavior low key, no one really will pay much attention to what you are eating or not eating. Naturally, some adaptations to social situations are called for, but a surprising percentage of the time, you can eat to suit your own special needs.

Examples

If you're hungry for breakfast at ten in the morning, see if you can arrange a break at that hour. Bring something from home that's nourishing and sustaining, even if it takes a bit of preparation before you leave the house.

If your hungry time is 4:30 P.M., and your spouse comes home from work at seven, consider the possibility of having your major meal when you really want it, but saving a part of dinner, such as soup, a small salad, or dessert to have while you are sitting together.

If you are always hungry at 10:00 P.M., plan to have something appealing but light, like fruit, crackers, yogurt, or popcorn.

If the late afternoon is a low period for you, instead of reaching for a sweet or a diet drink, have a nourishing snack— some fruit, a few rice cakes and vegetable broth. This little meal will raise your efficiency level for the remainder of the day, and prevent overeating at dinnertime.

When my daughter came home from high school, she was always starving! Since most school lunch periods seem to be for socializing rather than for eating, 3:30 in the afternoon was her hungriest time of the day. At first we went the traditional milk and cookies route. But by dinner time her appetite was gone and she wasn't hungry. We devised a radical plan: The most nourishing meal I could prepare was waiting for her when she arrived at home. All the vegetables and healthy foods that kids sometimes reject had new appeal when presented at this time of peak hunger. She ate and enjoyed this good, solid meal, and still had plenty of opportunities for snacking later in the evening.

I used this same system one summer when my sons came home from day camp at around 4:00 P.M. Nutritious foods were right there on the table, and they were too hungry to look for substitutions. The old saying that "hunger is the best sauce" can be used to good advantage when trying to get kids to eat healthy foods. Follow their natural rhythms whenever you can.

3. What Do I Want?

What food does my body need and want at this moment? If I could eat anything in the world right now, what would it be?

Many people have a great deal of difficulty answering that question. Their first response is something like "whatever's around, I guess." Reestablishing contact with signals coming from the inside telling you what you really want is frustrating at first, because the signals are so faint. Overly sweet things, artificial flavorings, excess alcohol, and smoking have dulled their message. You have to peel away the layers of modern living to get to the inner core of your original animal-self, where body-wisdom lies.

After a period of eating a diet abundant in fresh fruits and vegetables, and more natural foods in general, your inner voice will grow stronger. This "body-wisdom" will guide you toward eating in a healthier way. You will also notice that when you are really physiologically hungry, you tend to want more basic foods. It is when you are vaguely interested, and not really empty, that "appetite" plays the strongest part, leading to less nutritious selections.

If you "sort of" feel like eating something, or find yourself with your hand on the refrigerator door, but you don't know what you want, STOP. You're probably not really hungry yet. Get a drink of water, and wait a few minutes. As true hunger gets stronger, feel it. Tell yourself that this sensation is going to be your primary reason for eating from now on.

Now, what is it you want to eat? Don't go back to the refrigerator and look around to see what's there. Start from inside yourself. Hear the message, and then act on it.

Most overweight people have repeatedly pushed thoughts

of food out of their minds, fearing that they are weak and "obsessed" because food images tease them constantly. Often, this preoccupation is the result of severely restrictive diets. They are just plain *hungry,* and survival instincts are urging them to go out and find sustenance.

Overweight people are surprised to learn that many thin people spend a great deal of time thinking about food—planning their next meal, thinking of the upcoming trip to the food store, planning ahead to avoid being in a situation where there is nothing that they really want to eat.

You too should allow thoughts of food to play in your mind. Food must be a source of pleasure for you as well as nourishment. Tune in to precisely what you want at this moment. Okay, let's get the jokes out of the way: "Are you kidding? All I'd eat is chocolate." Or, "I'd go for nothing but pizza."

But you know that's not true. Given unlimited freedom, you very well might eat three boxes of chocolates the first day (especially if for years chocolate was "forbidden" to you). How about the second day? Probably a salad would sound just right, and the sight of another box of candy would make you sick.

Reestablish trust in yourself as a healthy organism with its own inner wisdom, which will lead you to select what your body needs and wants at each moment.

"Cravings"

We all have observed in ourselves and others, strange, strong food cravings. A teenager I know must have an artichoke every day; a client reported a month-long need for grapes; a friend knows when she wants almonds on a particular morning, and definitely not walnuts.

I went through a garlic phase. I absolutely had to have many (!) cloves of raw garlic with my salad every night although I was fully aware of the social consequences of my habit. Strangely and inexplicably, about a year after it began, it was over. Now I have little interest in eating garlic, despite my knowledge of its many reported health benefits.

Granted, these reports are anecdotal, but I suspect that the body has reasons for these cravings, and I believe you should listen to your body whenever possible.

Shopping: How Choosing Works

It has always been a cardinal rule for dieters never to go to the market when they are hungry. With the caution that you stay in the healthy sections, I advise the opposite. Wander through the fruits, vegetables, and meat and fish departments when you are beginning to get hungry (perhaps on your way home from work). What "feels" right today? Yams? Eggplant? Fish? Bananas? Listen to the messages.

I know how hard this is to do if you must shop with young children, but since what you eat is so important, try to rearrange the schedule so that at least sometimes you can shop slowly, deliberately, and alone. The foods you pick will become a part of you and those you love. Allow yourself the time to choose them with care.

4. Do I Like It?

Does this food I am eating taste good to me, or am I eating it just because it's there?

Is it worth spending the calories on this? Whether it is a simple snack or a fancy meal, you **are** spending calories and should get maximum pleasure from everything you eat. If an apple is mushy and has brown spots, trash it! If the restaurant meal is only fair, send it back, or swish it around with your fork to be polite, and plan to eat something wonderful later on. There is other, better food in the world, and you deserve the best.

When you make the choice to eat a high-calorie treat, it has nothing to do with "cheating." Cheating is by definition an underhanded act, so you tend to gobble food down indiscriminately without taking the time to savor it, as though you might be "caught in the act." But when you have *chosen* to indulge in a special food, the act is lifted from the cloudy realm of emotions into the light of adult reason. Enjoyment then becomes the primary goal.

Fran, who manages a country and western band, was just learning to live the 80/20 eating style. She was afraid that the minute she was tempted with high-calorie foods, she would go out of control.

One evening she was invited to a "down home" barbeque. When the buffet was served, she took her time looking over all the offerings. Her tastes had changed over the months she had been steadily losing weight. She was surprised that the barbequed ribs looked fatty and unappealing. Baked beans, cole slaw, raw vegetables and sourdough bread were the remainder of the fare, topped off by home-made pecan pie. Fran opted to go heavy on the vegetables and sourdough and have a little of the beans and cole slaw. But she decided that the pie had her name written on it, and this was her moment to indulge.

When she told this story in our behavior modification class, the other participants were enthralled as she described in detail taking that slice of pie over to a table away from everybody, eating it very slowly, and enjoying each delicious bite. She even cleared her palate several times with ice water.

"Didn't you want more?" someone asked. "No, I really didn't," she answered, "maybe because I ate it slowly, and knew I could have more if I wanted to."

"What would have happened if you used your will-power and stayed away from the pie all through the party?" I asked. "Oh," she laughed. "I would have stopped off at Marie Callender's Pie Shop on the way home, bought a whole pie, and eaten it in the car!"

5. Am I Full?

Am I full? Have I had enough? Am I continuing to eat just because it tastes good or because I think I should eat until it's all gone?

Many people really don't understand these questions. They simply continue to eat until all the food is gone. A client named Al couldn't figure out how or why people stop at two doughnuts when there are twelve in a box.

What does it mean to be full? Picture your stomach, an organ about the size of a fist, that expands to hold about one quart. Stuffing it beyond its capacity reduces its efficiency at processing food in preparation for passage to the small intestine. Eating to excess does not really produce more pleasure, but may cause indigestion and distress. It is definitely not a loving thing to do to yourself.

In some cultures, it is customary for participants at a festive meal to pat their stomachs in mock (or real) discomfort, claiming that the food was so good, no one could help but overeat. Rethink this custom! Food can be enjoyed and the cook complimented without suffering gastric distress and carrying home the souvenir of added pounds.

Just as the case of uncovering true hunger, it takes time and practice to get to know what proper fullness really feels like. To achieve this goal, I will not ask you to try techniques that nobody ever does for very long, like putting your fork down after every bite, or chewing each morsel a certain number of times.

I do recommend that before you have discovered the right amounts for you to eat, serve yourself a reasonable portion, and stop when it's gone. Tune in to how you feel. Was that enough? Do you only want more because it "tastes so good?" An old wives' tale says "Stop eating when the first burp surfaces." You may not feel full at that point, but at least pay attention to the signal.

It may be hard for you, but sometimes leave one or two bites on the plate, marking your official resignation from the clean-plate club. Thin people often stop eating foods they have really enjoyed while some still remains. Overweight people look in wonder at this phenomenon. How did "Slim" over there do that? How did he know *when* to do that? Give yourself time, and you too will know when you've had enough, just as you did when you were a baby.

We now know that it takes about twenty minutes for the "satiety center" in the brain to register fullness. Eating too fast doesn't give this mechanism a chance to go into action before too large a quantity has been consumed. So do slow down. You'll get more pleasure from what you eat, and the bonus of this behavior change will be to let you hear the increased volume of a vital, protective body signal.

Signals from Without

There are many OUTSIDE pressures urging us to eat:

• Fast-food restaurants with flashing neon signs and enticing memories.

• The proliferation of chocolate, cookie and ice cream concessions in shopping malls and neighborhoods.

• Advertising: the never-ending barrage of food stimuli.

• Friends and relatives who have hidden agendas, which may include the desire to keep you fat. These food-pushers can be friends, hosts, mothers, or mates.

• Holiday pressures to eat traditional, fattening foods.

• Buffets and all-you-can-eat meals, where it seems "wasteful" not to eat a lot.

Many overweight people make decisions about what, when, and how much to eat on the basis of these external cues. A tempting pastry in the bakery window is reason enough to eat, without consulting the body's state of hunger at the moment. This breakdown in intrabody communication is a common reason for people to gain weight.

Some researchers believe that food is metabolized more efficiently—used up—when eaten in response to true hunger. The digestive system seems more ready to do the job. When eating occurs at other times, fat may be stored more easily.

Become aware of the times you have eaten for external reasons, having nothing to do with body needs. It's time to reposition the eating control center to a spot *inside* of you. Becoming in tune with internal cues is a major behavior change that takes time and patience to achieve. I promise you that when the system is working, and you are back in harmony with your body's needs and rhythms, at last you will have discovered the one eating system that will never let you down.

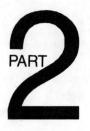

PART 2 the Process

4

Your Ideal Weight

For Life

Forget Dieting

The depth and degree of the problem of overweight in this country is disturbing: one out of three people are on some kind of diet at any particular time, and that number rises to two out of three for women. Eighty percent of women have been on a diet by age eighteen; 70% of girls under twelve are concerned about being fat. Most significant of all is that 95% of those who lose weight gain all or some of it back.

Anorexia and bulimia, unfamiliar conditions until very recently, are now common words. The manufacture and sale of diet pills is a huge industry. The typical outcome of this endless quest for a thin body is the "yo-yo syndrome"—repeatedly losing and then regaining weight. Most experts agree that maintaining a consistent level of obesity is healthier than repeatedly losing and gaining.

Extreme measures, such as of an inflatable "gastric bubble" placed in the stomach to create a feeling of fullness, actually sound appealing to surprising numbers of people. They apparently feel powerless to deal with food on a normal, rational basis.

People are so desperate to find an answer to the problem of being fat, they often abandon reason and grasp at almost any scheme—no matter how bizarre. When the latest diet craze appears, people rush to try it, each assuring the other that this one really works. "My friend lost ten pounds in five days, and all you eat is watermelon." Or "This one's great; you get to eat lots and lots of heavy cream." Substitute any absurd combination that comes to mind, and you won't be far off the mark. In fact, it seems that the more odd the diet, the stronger its appeal. The very strangeness and perceived originality ignites the false hope that this plan is truly different; here at last is the secret food, the ultimate combination, the magic potion that will be "it"—that will make the pounds melt away effortlessly.

Usually the prescription is the adherence to some variation of a very low-calorie program. Clients have reported to me that sometimes they face Monday morning's severely restrictive diet with a feeling that punishment is what they deserve for past "sins" of weakness and over-indulgence. Suffering deprivation, therefore, is a kind of penance, offering absolution for the week-end's transgressions.

I have seen strict deprivation diets create what I call a "snarling mentality." One bite of a "forbidden food" leads inevitably to a binge. And why not? A voice inside says, "Quick, while we have the chance, devour it all! Who knows what new ridiculous scheme we will be starting tomorrow."

No one stays on these diets very long. The weight loss is rapid, but so is the regain. With each returning pound comes the heavier burden of feelings of failure, guilt, and inadequacy. "What's wrong with me? Why am I so weak? Why can't I solve this problem once and for all?"

The saddest cases I have seen were very obese people who had been put on some sort of fasting program at a university, or by a "diet doctor," and had lost large amounts of weight. When they gain the pounds back (and often more), they are convinced that they are total failures. Their painful conclusion is "If those experts can't help me, I must be beyond hope."

One beautiful young actress told me that she enjoyed being at her goal weight for "one brief shining moment." It lasted three days before the spike back up began. When the weight started to come back, she didn't know what to do. Like so many others, she knew everything about dieting, and nothing about healthful eating.

Making It Even Harder for Yourself

Repeatedly adhering to very low-calorie diets, and frequently skipping meals has been shown to utterly sabotage the frustrated dieter. Because the body adapts to what it perceives as a threat of possible starvation by *lowering* the basal metabolic rate (the rate at which we burn calories) to conserve energy, getting off the diet treadmill becomes increasingly difficult. Feelings of lethargy make you tend to stay still. The last thing you feel like doing is being active, which of course is the best way to burn calories. As with a hibernating animal, all processes slow down while your precious fat is conserved. Since its food supply has been curtailed, the body's mechanisms send messages to **increase** the appetite. We must have nourishment to survive; therefore the brain and body try to propel us to go out and forage the way any animal would do under such circumstances. No wonder perpetual dieters describe being obsessed with thoughts of food. Your body is doing what comes naturally—attempting to survive. Trying to battle the force of this life-sustaining hunger drive makes you uncomfortable all day long. In the end, hunger will win.

You might try to commit suicide by holding your breath, but inevitably survival instincts will take over, and you'll breathe. In the same way, you can put yourself on a starvation regimen, but eventually your biological instincts will take over and you will eat.

Losing Weight Too Fast Is Counterproductive

On crash diets that produce rapid weight loss (most often with no exercise), it is mostly muscle tissue that is broken down, not the targeted fat stores. When weight is quickly regained, the same amount of lean tissue is not restored. Instead, the proportion of fat tissue to lean muscle mass goes to higher and higher levels. <u>It is important to know that only muscle tissue burns fat.</u> The more lean muscle tissue you have, the more calories you burn each day, and the more you can eat without gaining weight. Sadly, some dieters have so increased the proportion of fat in their bodies that they can eat very little and still not lose weight.

The body is so wise. It assumes (usually with justification) that since it has faced starvation once, it had better prepare for this eventuality again. It somehow learns to store fat even more efficiently with each crash diet. This brilliant biological adaptation makes losing weight more and more difficult each time you try. The net result is that the poor, suffering, well-intentioned dieter (whose periodic displays of will-power astonish his or her slim friends) seems to gain weight faster and lose it slower than someone who has never before dieted.

The Choosing Not Cheating Plan Is For Life

The Choosing Not Cheating Plan is very different in that it does not severely restrict food intake. Women should eat no less than 1,200 calories a day; men no less than 1,500. In fact, there is no need to count calories at all. The CNC Plan does not promise quick, dramatic weight loss in time for your wedding, vacation, or the up-coming-bathing-suit season. How much weight you lose by next month is really insignificant when you think about it in terms of a lifetime. Naturally your aim is to get down to the weight you want to be. But what really matters is that once you do, you know how to stay there *permanently* and *comfortably*.

Since the goal is to lose fat, not "weight," which includes bone, water and muscle, you will see a slower reduction on the scale than quick weight-loss schemes produce. But you will be losing what you want to lose—**FAT.** Experience has also shown you that the quicker the loss, the quicker the regain. This time do it right: the slow, steady way that lasts. Don't put yourself through the distress of "dieting" or being a "yo-yo" ever again.

Because I want you to adopt a long-range perspective, I urge you not to get on the scale more frequently than once a month—a radical idea for many experienced dieters. A daily weigh-in does not take into account normal bodily fluctuations, like hormonal states, the fullness of the digestive tract, and various fluid balances. Besides, the scale is an inaccurate measure of **fat** loss. A better indicator is an article of clothing that will begin to fit differently as your body's proportions change to more muscle and less fat. You really do lose inches, and look more fit and "tight" instead of flabby. (Of course you are pursuing your exercise program—a vital part of the plan. (See Chapter 6.)

When you weigh yourself every day, you give great power to the mechanical device on your bathroom floor. It becomes the arbiter of your success or failure. Sometimes not losing weight on a day when you had expected to can propel you into out-of-control eating on the grounds that "no matter what I do, nothing works anyway."

Most important, frequent trips to the scale (Some people perform the ritual two or three times in twenty-four hours!) reinforces the erroneous concept that successful weight management is measured on a daily basis. In reality, the ultimate measures of your accomplishments are: Did you reach and maintain your goal weight? Are your tastes changing so that you are **enjoying** new, low-calorie, low-fat foods? Do you have a normal, comfortable relationship with food which allows you to "party" when the time is right, and then go right back to your healthier, low-calorie way of eating?

Where Is the "Diet?"

The route to the goals described above is not to be found in any one-size-fits-all printed diet, and so you won't find one here. Here's why:

• The minute you have something to go "on," some day, some month, you must go "off." Going "off" implies a return to your old eating patterns—guaranteed to bring back your old body.

• When each detail is spelled out for you, you feel you are "being taken care of." The burden of responsibility for making decisions about which foods to choose, and in what amounts is the diet-writer's, not yours. It is a childlike position, and probably not the way you like to be treated in other aspects of your life. Choices made from within are the ones that will last, and are different from those imposed by someone else.

• Diets have frequently been described as a crutch. In the case of a broken leg, a crutch offers support only while bones are mending. The diet mentality encourages the use of one crutch or another on a continuing basis. The result is that you never learn to walk confidently and independently on your own.

• Having a printed diet is like visiting a foreign country with a translator as your companion. As long as this knowledgeable person is by your side, you run into no difficulty. But what if you are suddenly lost and alone? How much better it would have been if you had learned the language of this new place before you left home.

• The most compelling reason of all: How could I tell you that Monday's lunch should be a lamb chop and a salad, when that day you really want to eat a turkey sandwich? A primary, necessary goal of this program is to reawaken your own internal body signals, which will, in time, reliably tell you when your body is truly physiologically hungry, what it needs and wants at that moment, and when you have had enough and should stop eating. If I place my printed diet between you and these cues, regardless of how healthy the foods are, I would be offering just another short-term solution to a long-term problem. A Chinese proverb says, "Give a man a fish, and you feed him for a day; teach a man to fish, and you've fed him for a lifetime." Let's learn how to fish.

Lose Weight by "Playing Percentages"

I won't give you a printed diet, but I will tell you how to lose weight using the Choosing Not Cheating "80/20" system—a livable program that puts YOU in control of the amount of weight you lose, and how fast you lose it.

The "80%" is a flexible number, representing your "normal" way of eating—your **home base foods.** Eighty percent of the foods you eat will be those that give you the highest nutrition for the lowest caloric expenditure.

The "20%" refers to the festive foods—those you choose to eat just for fun. You decide when the time, situation, and foods are right for you to spend the extra calories.

The percentage of the time you will be eating in each style is up to you. If you are pleased with your current weight, an 80/20 percent formula might be just right: about 80% of the food you eat will be low-calorie, high nutrition selections—primarily complex carbohydrates—and about 20% of your eating will be "partying"—whatever that means for you.

If you want to lose weight as quickly as possible, you might be tempted to stay in a low-fat, low calorie mode 100% of the time until you reach your goal. **ALL** the foods you eat would be vegetables, fruits, grains, and legumes, with the addition of small quantities of the leanest fish, poultry, and meats. You would eat no additional fats of any kind, no sugar, white flour products, and no processed foods. You would emphasize raw and lightly cooked vegetables, fresh fruits, bulky cereals and grains, potatoes, and some legumes.

You would make a commitment to exercise aerobically at least 5 days a week in addition to **moving** your body every day—take walks, take the stairs, not the elevator, etc.

You can be sure that if you follow this program, you will lose weight, feel vibrant, and probably be healthier than you've ever been. As you see your weight go down and your energy level go up, you become more and more convinced of the wisdom of following humankind's original diet consisting of whole, natural unprocessed fruits, vegetables, grains and legumes, supplemented with lean animal protein. I recommend that you select from these natural foods **most of the time.**

But even though you want to drop those excess pounds as quickly as possible, I don't advise you to attempt to remain rigidly in this spartan mode, denying yourself all "festive" eating and special occasions for any appreciable length of time. Such resolutions invariably lead to failure.

Life doesn't come to a screeching halt just because you've decided you want to be lean. To achieve ultimate success, you must deal with reality. You will still have social functions, business lunches, celebratory dinners to attend. There will continue to be moments when you feel the need for a special treat, when your usual healthy foods just won't do.

For this reason a 90/10, or 80/20 percent program is much more realistic, and stands a greater chance of producing long-term success. Experience has shown that when people feel deprived, it's only a matter of time before they rebel. Going for months without having dessert, eating something just for fun, or eating something just because it tastes good tends to explode in a cataclysmic binge. You cannot put your life on hold. You must continue to **live** while you are on the road to your goal weight. Like so much in life, the process is no less important than the product.

You are firmly committed to becoming fit, and staying that way for the rest of your life. However, because you are seeing things in long-range terms and not seeking a quick-fix, your flexible attitude allows you to make *situational* choices about what eating style is right for you at any particular time.

Your "Balance Point"

Here are the criteria you should consider in finding your own "balance point"—what your percentages should be: How motivated (always within the bounds of sound nutrition) are you to lose the extra fat? How much time and effort are you willing to put into exercise? What's going on in your life right now—socially, emotionally, at work, in your family? Are you about to leave on a long-planned vacation? Are you under emotional stress?

Examples of "Playing the Percentages"

Jim, an aspiring actor, had decided to keep his calories and fats low, increase his exercise, and at last get down to his best weight. He hoped this might help him get the acting parts he wanted.

He was doing very well from Monday to Friday, enjoying those healthy fruits, vegetables and grains, feeling energized, and very pleased with himself.

Unexpectedly, an old friend from his Off-Broadway days arrived from New York, and asked Jim and some others to a reunion dinner at a pizzeria. Jim had these options:

1. Decline the dinner invitation, afraid to go "off his diet," miss the opportunity to renew old friendships, and have a great evening.

2. Go, but explain that he is on a diet (automatically making everyone else feel uncomfortable and inhibited), order a plain salad with no dressing, pass up the beer or wine, and stare down that pizza with a ferocious surge of will-power.

Either course of action would likely be followed by a solitary binge at home, eating anything available, good-tasting or not, or by a late-night trip to the store for six candy bars, a quart of ice cream, and a whole frozen cake.

Such a predictable outcome is the direct result of enduring deprivation, especially in public. Feeling different, less adequate in dealing with food, somehow inferior to the others who are allowed to "go to the party," sets the stage for eating many times more calories than a slice or two of pizza would have contained.

3. Shift into a more flexible mode—his "festive" 10 or 20%. Enjoy a reasonable portion of pizza. Eat it slowly and with delight, because he is not "cheating" but choosing. Jim would have no need to grab for the last few slices on the platter in anticipation of Monday morning's remorse and new diet. He knows that pizza will always be there for him whenever he chooses to spend the calories and that it will feel as right to get back to his fresh, whole, low-calorie foods tomorrow as it did to enjoy this splurge tonight.

Times of Tension

A word about those typical pressures of living: While periods of tension and transition are not ideal times to deprive yourself of your usual foods, it is important to understand the futility of waiting until life is free of tension and stress before embarking on a weight-reduction program. Of course, that moment of serenity never comes. Remember that thin people have problems too, but at your ideal weight ("fighting weight"), you somehow feel better able to cope with any situation, difficult person, or eventuality. So you may as well get started now!

No matter what percentage formula you choose, you know that at any point, you have "permission" to eat anything you want. You are released from the extremes of the "on-a-diet" or "eating-out-of-control" mentality. You start to think like a slim person, knowing that a high-calorie meal or day is just part of living the Good Life and does not signal your downfall.

You know too that you never have to give up any foods *forever*, unless you find that some foods have lost their appeal, and you choose not to eat them anymore. I reject the idea that there are foods you must banish permanently from your life because they are "too fattening." I overheard two rather plump women scanning the menu at the Polo Lounge of the Beverly Hills Hotel. One said with a sigh, "Well, I guess there are some things you can just never eat if you want to be thin."

I don't accept that point of view for myself or for you. I refuse to go through life forever telling a great chef to "hold the sauce." Chocolate, ice cream and fettucini must play some part in my present and future *but only a judicious percentage of the time.* You and I are both capable of controlling that percentage so that we can have good health, a slim body, and the fun and pleasure of eating. We **CAN** have it all.

One critical decision must be made: not to continue to overeat at some point just because you've "blown it anyway." Having a piece of cake at a birthday party because it felt just right at the moment must not lead to stopping on the way home for a pizza. The birthday cake was the chosen indulgence of a non-dieting, rational adult who gets to join in life's celebrations. "Dieting" and "pigging out" are not your only choices. There is also the rational, balanced, slim person's approach to food.

If you were standing on the edge of a cliff and your foot slipped, your response wouldn't be, "Oh well, I'm halfway over I might as well go the whole way." Instead, you would step back to more solid ground. You must learn to do this with food as well.

In this case, your "solid ground" is the 80%—your high-nutrition, low calorie style of eating.

Wendy, a paralegal, and her attorney-husband are about to leave for a two week vacation in France. Her long-range goal is to lose fat, but she doesn't want to think about it while she's away.

This circumstance is not as difficult as it seems. Most people do not actually gain the weight they fear when out of town, but rather when they are at home with continuous access to the refrigerator, second helpings, and snacks.

Wendy's first consideration should be to plan for lots of walking, and all the other exercise she can work in. Then she should decide that while she will not deprive herself of memorable dining experiences, neither will she "go crazy." She knows that too many high-fat cheeses, croissants, and patés are really too "expensive" calorically. Sometimes she will have only fruits or salads, because after having enjoyed some very rich meals, her internal signals will guide her to those choices.

To go on a vacation and try to stay on a strict diet (unless medical conditions demand it), or to make a fuss about the subject to yourself or your traveling companions is, to my mind, sinful! But it is a more grievous sin to abuse the body by stuffing it with high calorie foods, just because "now's my chance to pig-out." That kind of thinking is no longer acceptable to anyone who sees the overview, who looks at food with a sense of balance, and who has a life-time eating plan on which to rely.

Getting the Value You Deserve

Since your choices are always situational, and you are free of the extremes of either dieting or eating out-of-control, you will get into the routine of continually asking yourself, "Is this really worth it?" You will become very choosy about what is good enough for you to eat. This concept applies equally to seeking the perfect pear and selecting the best three-star restaurant.

One Monday morning at the gym, I was riding the exercise bicycle next to a woman named Karen, who is an accountant for many well-known people in the record business. We chatted about our weekend's activities, and I told her in glowing terms about my special anniversary dinner at Spago, currently one of the most popular restaurants in Los Angeles.

I described the delicious sourdough French bread, perfect salad, seafood pasta in a creamy sauce, and just about the best dessert I had ever had—their famous macadamia nut tart with homemade caramel ice cream.

Karen knew I was a diet counselor, and looked at me skeptically. "You really ate that?" she asked. I assured her that I did, and that in this case, the dinner was so delicious that I surely got full value for the calories spent. "Oh," she said, "I guess you must starve yourself all week, and then go crazy on weekends, right?"

Wrong! That is a dangerous, misguided, all-to-frequent pattern followed by perennial fat-fighters. Sure, you're more likely to enjoy festive occasions on weekends, because that's when you tend to be with other people. Thankfully there **ARE** festive occasions in people's lives and weekends are the usual time to celebrate them.

But what if you have nothing special to do on Friday night? Do you overeat indiscriminately because "damn it, I've earned it. I've been 'good' all week?" I hope not.

You know that special foods will always be there. You just choose the times and the situations that you really want them. And any occasions that you're perfectly content with simple, healthy foods is just a plus in your column. (Remember, the conversation about dinner at Spago was while **exercising**–using up those delicious calories is part of the balance.)

Sometimes a planned "festive" occasion never materializes. Jane, a prominent charity fund-raiser, looks forward to lunch with friends at a lovely garden-patio restaurant, where the pastry chef is reputed to be excellent. But when her dessert arrives, it turns out to be mediocre. After a bite or two, she makes no comment, but puts her fork down, thinking of better ways to spend those calories. In other words, while disappointed that this particular experience is less than anticipated, she begins to plan the extra good dinner she might have, or even the special fudge brownie she could buy at the shop next door.

Yes, that moment when you choose to stop eating a dessert, or any food, is difficult and new, but the important concept is that you are too **SPECIAL** to eat anything just because it's there. "Because it's there" may be reason enough to climb Mt. Everest, but it should not be sufficient cause to eat anything mediocre. You spend the same number of calories on a cold, greasy cheeseburger as one sizzling hot from the grill. The stale cookies at the back of the cupboard "cost" the same as chewy, warm ones just out of the oven.

You need to gobble down inferior foods for two reasons only: the threat of impending starvation, or the frantic need to eat anything that will become a forbidden food on next Monday's diet. Probably, starvation is not your concern. I hope "dieting" isn't either.

Special Times

There are times in your life that are very social, very special, conducive to a lot of higher-calorie eating: the holiday season, a tour of France, Italy, Hong Kong . . ., the weeks before a large wedding, a cruise. But there are also times when its easy to keep your eating simple and low-fat—when your social life is quiet, and few demands are placed upon you—when spartan eating is appropriate, and doesn't feel like deprivation. These opportunities should be seized as a time to "bank" some calories, perhaps to get to your leanest weight in anticipation of future events at which you will want to indulge in some gala eating.

· ·

Elaine was shooting a movie on location on a tropical island. She was under pressure, very busy and the heat wilted her appetite. She decided that the time, far away from her usual hectic social life back in Los Angeles, offered the perfect opportunity for a "cleansing" regimen.

Most of the food wasn't very good, but the local fruits were spectacular! There was a feast of exotic varieties: mangos, papayas, pineapples, bananas, and some she had never seen before. She supplemented this luscious fresh fruit diet with the plain rice the locals ate, some greens and other vegetables, and occasionally some broiled fish.

The film was not a great success, but Elaine looks back nostalgically on that time of natural eating. She lost a few pounds, and remembers that she never felt better in her life.

. . . .

Jennifer was spending a few weeks at home before returning to college in the fall. She welcomed the time to do some shopping, reading, and relaxing in anticipation of the busy year coming up. Although she occasionally went out for a light meal, she was grateful for the opportunity to eat in a healthy, low-fat, rather spartan style, and to drop a few pounds in the bargain. To live that way forever? Unthinkable. But for this limited span of time, it was a welcome, positive break.

Many people report a powerful feeling of "being in control" when there is a period of very healthy, low-calorie eating. When you know you're taking good care of yourself, you like the way you feel. Perhaps this is the reason that health spas are more popular today than ever before. For a few days or weeks, you are taught by experts how to live a healthy, positive lifestyle, eating nutritiously and paring off excess pounds.

People do well at spas, and most follow the "diet" religiously, not only because they want to lose weight and get in shape, but also because they know that the program won't last forever. You can create this atmosphere and outlook for yourself *at home*. Treat your 80% time as though you were a guest at a health spa, but one who always has the option of "taking a trip into town."

Do I Have to Count Calories?

Are fatty foods more "fattening?"
Calorie knowledge is a useful tool for achieving a slim body. But new data are causing us to look at some basic ideas in the field of weight control.

It was once accepted as a fundamental principle that a calorie is a calorie; that 100 calories of zucchini and 100 calories of chocolate may differ in volume, but that they act the same when eaten. Once you eat more calories than you burn, the excess is stored as fat, regardless of the original source.

Now, in research including that of Elliot Danforth of the University of Vermont and Jean-Pierre Flatt at the University of Massachussetts Medical Center in Worcester, some important new hypotheses have emerged. The indications are that calories from fat are more "fattening" than those from protein or carbohydrate. Dietary fat (fatty foods you eat), being closer to body fat chemically, must go through fewer complicated changes before it is stored at such depots as hips, thighs, and abdomen. Carbohydrates, on the other hand, when eaten in excess, are stored in relatively small quantities as glycogen in the liver and muscles (Barnett: 1986; Liebman: 1989).

When laboratory animals were fed *the same number of calories,* those on a high fat diet gained more weight than those on a lower fat diet (Barnett: 1986; Liebman: 1989). In addition, it was discovered that a high carbohydrate diet seems to stimulate metabolism in the same way that exercise does (but to a lesser extent), so that more calories are burned (Barnett: 1986; Liebman: 1989). These data may explain why it is easier to lose weight on a high complex-carbohydrate diet, even when large quantities of foods are eaten.

Do I Have to Study Calorie Charts?

While you don't have to count calories, you do have to know something about the relative "cost" of food. Selecting food without a minimum knowledge of calories is like tossing unpriced items into your shopping cart. When you get to the check-out counter, you may find that you have done serious damage to your budget.

It's also important to have a good idea of the content of what you eat so you can be wary of empty calories—those foods and beverages which are nutritionally worthless, yet contain lots of calories—like refined sugar, soft drinks, and alcohol. As you reduce your over-all caloric consumption on your way to being slim, it is vital to get the maximum nutritional mileage out of each food calorie. As they say in the Defense Department, you want to get the "biggest bang for your buck."

So do buy a reliable calorie book. (I recommend *Calorie Guide to Brand Names and Basic Foods* by Barbara Kraus, published by New American Library, and available in paperback.) Use it as a reference to help you make intelligent, informed decisions. But don't be a slave to it. Some of the fattest people I know are calorie experts. They can eyeball a portion of anything, and come up with an accurate number, but that skill alone has not been of much help in controlling their weight.

On the other hand, some of my beginning clients are "virgin dieters"—they know absolutely nothing about the calorie or fat content of any food. These are usually people who were always thin, and then put on weight during or following a life change like having a baby, suddenly being unable to exercise, or reaching middle age.

For these beginners, I recommend a quick dose of awareness. Their assignment is to write down every bit of food they eat; compute the portion size; (What does four ounces of fish look like on a plate? How big is a six ounce apple?) look up and record the calories. They are invariably surprised by some of the totals, especially of foods they've always eaten, but aren't even crazy about. "Potato chips have that many calories?" (1800 per twelve ounce bag). In the process of your research, you might be surprised to learn just how high in fat and calories certain foods really are. You may find many of them aren't worth the expense. An eight ounce slice of rib roast with all visible fat removed, a fast-food very-crisp chicken dinner with all the trimmings, or a cup of mixed nuts total nearly 1,000 calories each, close to the total daily requirement for a small woman!

Conversely, computing the number of calories you've eaten sometimes eases a guilty conscience. Often foods that felt sinful going down turn out to be lower in calories than they tasted.

One day while out for a walk, I got into conversation with a lovely, slim girl named Jeanne. Hearing about my work, she immediately launched into a "confession" of the previous night's "bad" behavior. She said that on the way home from the office she felt a special craving for frozen yogurt with apple topping. She indulged herself, but she didn't have dinner. When we computed the calories of that "terrible binge," she was surprised to learn that the number was about 300. By adding up the remainder of her day's calories, we found the number to be quite moderate. Plus she had gone for that long walk.

Certainly I do not advocate a dinner of such low nutritional value very often, but by knowing the calorie cost of foods, plans can be made for lower calorie choices at the next meal or for the next day.

In the past you might have been one of those who rigorously measured and weighed small quantities of food in your efforts to lose weight. (How many times have you scooped exactly ½ cup of cottage cheese, or weighed a handful of ground beef?) Like so many others, you probably found this approach to be ineffective in the long run. There is nothing wrong with your measuring skills or your will power. The fault lies not in the dieter, but in the philosophy of continuous deprivation, and in the *content* of the diet. Attempting to eat small quantities of high-fat and/or low-fiber foods will not work for very long.

Without permission to enjoy life sometimes, without the feelings of satisfaction produced by a full stomach, no weighing, measuring, or counting can carry you through the tough times. Yes, know about calories. But to achieve and maintain your ideal weight, know that sometimes you're going to eat foods that add up to big numbers, and that's okay. Most important, make the high-nutrition, high-fiber, filling foods which you will learn about in the following chapters your "normal," baseline way of eating.

5

Choosing Meals

Since other people's formulas have probably let you down, it's time for you to take control of your body. Regard any piece of paper as absurd when it tells you, a unique individual, what, when, and how to perform one of life's most basic functions: eating. Choose never to go "on" or "off" another packaged program. Choose never to give up control for the rest of your life.

Shape your personal eating plan from a wide variety of the healthy foods listed below; tailoring your plan to suit your own needs and tastes. Call upon your increasingly strong and reliable internal cues to tell you what your body wants and needs at a particular time. Make your plan flexible enough to accommodate the times of festivity—the only way you will achieve permanent success.

There are no rules about what you must eat each day or at a particular meal. Physiological hunger will be your guide to quantity as well as specific food selection. Many people who have lost touch with their inner hunger and fullness signals find such freedom disconcerting at first, and are skeptical that the method can work. They are more comfortable being told to eat a cup of this, or four ounces of that, fearful that if they are given freedom, they will never stop eating.

These fears are unfounded, as long as you remember that it is fats of all kind that make you fat. Sometimes in the beginning, people **DO** tend to overeat formerly forbidden foods like sweet fruits, potatoes, and cereals. But once the realization takes hold that this plan is forever—no new "diet" will take away these good, wholesome foods—more moderate eating just happens naturally. You are no longer victim to the "snarling mentality," eating everything you can before the opportunity is gone and the next "diet" begins.

The majority of what you eat, your "home-base" foods, will be those which provide the highest nutrition for the lowest amount of fat. Following is a list of suggestions and possibilities to assist you. Use these guidelines to formulate a shopping list, and give you some menu ideas.

Be creative! Breakfast, lunch and dinner foods can be freely intermixed. Try something new like a turkey sandwich for breakfast, a yam (hot or cold) for lunch, oatmeal and a banana for dinner. Leftover whole grains, vegetables, potatoes, or squash are all excellent for any meal or snack.

Discuss the Plan with Your Doctor

At about this point in every book about losing weight, the author warns you to consult your physician before embarking on this or any other diet. Please do so if you are a pregnant or lactating woman, or if you have any other limiting health problems.

Since this program advocates returning to humankind's original way of eating, and never dropping below 1,200 calories per day for women, or 1,500 calories per day for men, this program can hardly be labeled a "diet." However, discussing the plan with a doctor can be beneficial. His or her support for this health-enhancing way of eating might give you an added boost of motivation.

In addition, monitoring your blood pressure, cholesterol and triglyceride levels, and probably watching them improve will show you convincingly that by eating in this high complex-carbohydrate, low-fat style, you are not only getting slim and more attractive on the outside, but markedly helping your body be healthier on the inside.

Breakfast Suggestions

Whole fruits (preferable to juice). Pick the best of the season.

Whole grain hot cereals with no fat, sugar, or preservatives.
Examples: oatmeal, oat bran, Wheatena, Roman Meal, Cream of Wheat, cracked wheat, Ralston.

Whole grain cold cereals with no fat, sugar, or preservatives
Examples: Grapenuts, Shredded Wheat, Nutri-grain, Kashi*, puffed grains, Uncle Sam, Oatios, Oat Bran Crunch, any of the Health Valley brand cereals, including Oat Bran Flakes, Amaranth Flakes, 7 Grain Sprouted Flakes. Swiss style muesli (Familia) is very nutritious, but even the kind without added sugar has additional calories from nuts and raisins.

Cooked grains, such as brown rice, barley, millet, Kashi*, kasha, corn.

Sprouted grains. Sprouted wheat is easiest to find in some produce sections, or sprout your own wheat or rye berries (the whole grain kernel).

Whole grain bread, toast, crackers or muffins, made with little or no fat or sugar.

Non-fat whole grain English Muffins

Whole grain pancakes, made without fat or sugar.

Whole wheat pita bread.

Whole wheat Chapati (a kind of flat, tortilla-like Indian bread).

Rice cakes.

Whole wheat matzo.

Unleavened, dense loaves (Essen Breads).

---

*Kashi, an excellent multi-grain product, comes in 2 forms: a hot cooked cereal or side dish, and a cold cereal.

Corn tortillas (not fried).

Wheat germ (in moderation, because it's relatively high in calories—but a tablespoon adds a lot of flavor and nutrition).

Non-fat (skimmed) milk.

Non-fat yogurt.

Low-fat cottage cheese, farmer cheese, or hoop cheese.

Jams, jellies and spreads (like apple butter) made from fruit only, no sugar.

Eggs poached, boiled or cooked in a non-stick pan. If you enjoy eggs, have them only occasionally, and never if your cholesterol level is too high.

Possibilities for Lunch and Dinner

Whole fruits, fresh fruit salad.

Vegetables of any kind, raw or steamed.

Salads of greens, any fresh vegetables, sprouts, with no-oil dressing, or very small amount of olive oil, depending on how low you want to keep your calorie count.

Baked potatoes, yams, sweet potatoes—all good hot or cold.

Cooked winter squash such as butternut, acorn, banana.

Cooked grains.
Examples: brown rice, barley, millet, Kashi.

Corn on the cob, or corn kernels without sauce or butter.

Whole grain bread, pita, crackers, muffins, or matzo, made with little or no fat or sugar.

Low-fat cottage cheese, farmer cheese, or hoop cheese.

Non-fat yogurt (add your own fruit, or have it with cut up vegetables or a salad.

Soups and clear broths made without fat, such as bean, vegetable, barley, gazpacho, bouillion.

Tofu.

Ramen (Japanese-style noodles and broth. Check sodium content if that's a problem for you.)

Cooked beans or legumes.
Examples: black beans, lima beans, pinto beans, great northerns, garbanzos (chick peas), kidney beans, split peas, lentils.

Sprouted beans or lentils.

Vegetarian combinations.
Examples: rice and beans, corn or flour tortillas and beans, lima beans and barley, all made without oil and not fried.

Mashed potatoes fluffed with non-fat milk.

Pasta in any form, with a low fat sauce.

Ratatouille and other vegetable stews.

Grilled, baked, or barbequed vegetables.

(Remember: It is recommended that all animal protein be limited. If and when you choose to have meat, use it as a condiment, not as the centerpiece of the meal.)

Poached or broiled fish.

Shellfish, hot or cold.

Sushi, sashimi.

Tuna, water packed, no mayonnaise.

Sardines, mustard packed or remove oil, if oil packed.

Canned salmon, water packed.

Turkey or chicken, skin removed.

The leanest cuts of red meat, including flank, round, chuck, tenderloin, sirloin tip.

Sandwiches are fine (on whole grain bread or pita). Switch from mayonnaise to mustard. Ketchup, although most brands contain sugar, is still relatively low in calories. Have unlimited amounts of lettuce, tomato and sprouts on your sandwich if you like them.

Snack Ideas

Air-popped popcorn with no butter or oil.

Rice cakes, bread sticks, whole wheat matzo, or other whole grain, no fat, no sugar crackers.

Raw vegetables of all kinds.

Fresh fruits of all kinds.

Dried fruit (in moderation).

Fruit "leathers" without sugar.

Clear broth.

Ready-to-eat whole grain cereals.

Frozen fruit bars, with no sugar.

A Few Sample Days

Although you won't find specific directions about what foods to eat at particular times of the day, perhaps you will find it helpful to read about some choices made by others who have used and who are currently using the CNC Plan to be slim and healthy. This is how they eat in their "80%" mode, when they are keeping calories low, and nutrition high. Each person "parties" in his or her own special way. Eating in the low-calorie style most of the time is what allows them to enjoy those festive times freely.

REMINDER

When you are trying to keep your calories as low as possible, eliminate **fats** and **sugar** from your diet, and fill up on complex carbohydrates.

AVOID	EAT THESE FOODS
butter, oil, cheese, cream, whole milk, fried foods, bakery products, chips, processed foods, mayonnaise, red meat (beef, lamb, pork, ham, veal, hot dogs)	fruits vegetables grains legumes

• •

Sam plays racquetball before going to his law office. He showers and changes at his club, then stops off at a coffee shop near the office for breakfast. By this time the waitress knows that Sam has one-half grapefruit or melon, depending on the season, a bowl of oatmeal, and one slice of whole wheat bread, hold the butter, and decaffeinated coffee.

If he is eating lunch out with a client or friend, he chooses a restaurant where there are always salads on the menu, and has the dressing served on the side. Or, he opts for a local Sushi restaurant, currently a very popular choice in Southern California. If at his desk, he'll order a turkey sandwich with lettuce and mustard, and have it with a cup of instant vegetable broth.

Dinner is usually broiled fish or chicken without the skin, vegetables, salad and fresh fruit.

• •

Lynn writes at home. She has fruit and coffee before her morning walk. Her hungry time for breakfast is around 10:00 A.M., when she has whole grain cereal and a banana. Lunch is often one or two baked potatoes, which she enjoys while sitting at the typewriter.

She is a vegetarian, so dinner always starts with a large salad of greens and vegetables, and then usually lentils or beans and brown rice, or corn tortillas and pinto beans with salsa. She saves some fresh fruit for the times she gets hungry later in the evening.

• •

Lenore is an agent who is constantly rushed and under pressure. She has never been able to make time in the mornings for breakfast except for some fruit which she eats while dressing. On her way to work she stops for a bran muffin at a bakery that guarantees that the ingredients are 100% whole wheat flour, and a minimum of oil and honey. She enjoys the muffin at her desk, with a container of non-fat yogurt, and a pot of herb tea.

Lunch is often water-packed tuna and lettuce, on whole wheat pita, hastily put together in the office kitchen.

Sometimes when she gets home in the evening, she is so tense she has the need to feel "filled up." What seems to work is a large bowl of pasta with a tomato sauce made with no oil. Her cleaning lady is instructed to wash and slice raw vegetables so that Lenore can have something to munch on when she walks in the door. When the desire to snack overtakes her in the evenings, she makes a giant bowl of popcorn in her air-popper.

• •

Kathy had trouble learning to eat breakfast. She started with fruit, and then got used to crunchy whole-grain cold cereal, with yogurt, bran and some fruit on top. If she's too rushed at home, she assembles it in a plastic container, and eats it at her coffee break.

Lunch is very social in Kathy's business. Almost every day, she has a luncheon engagement at a restaurant. She will order such things as shrimp or crab cocktail, seafood salad with dressing on the side, or broiled fish. At a Chinese restaurant, she orders sautéed mixed vegetables and rice, or a shrimp and vegetable dish.

After eating in restaurants for lunch, dinner is usually very light—sometimes just fruit and non-fat yogurt, a baked potato, or some steamed vegetables and a few rice cakes.

• •

Jill is a Hollywood wife. (Yes, there are such creatures.) She feels driven to maintain her youthful figure, and has a standing appointment with a plastic surgeon. Much of her day is spent in taking care of herself, then making appearances at functions where it is important to be "seen."

Her personal trainer comes to the house three times a week for an exercise session, and on two other days there is an 11:00 A.M. tennis game.

Since so much eating is done in public where she never wants to appear less than naturally slim, her non-public meals are quite spartan. But she is convinced that the best nutrition makes her look her best, so she is extremely careful about what she eats.

Breakfast is usually one piece of eight-grain bread toasted, spread with a teaspoon of pure fruit jam, a small piece of fruit, and English Breakfast tea. Lunch is always assorted cut up vegetables in a large salad bowl, on a bed of arugula and other fancy greens. When she and her husband dine alone, they eat as simply as possible—broiled fish, brown rice, cooked vegetables, and bean sprouts.

• •

Every morning I start my day with a large (32 oz.) glass of room temperature water into which I squeeze the juice of one whole lemon. This ancient piece of folk wisdom has been followed by many people for years (some prefer to squeeze the lemon into a cup of hot water). I find it a cleansing and refreshing drink—a perfect way to wake up the digestive system. I then have one piece of fruit (melon, grapefruit, orange, papaya) before I go to the gym.

My "real" breakfast, which follows the morning workout, always consists of sprouted grains, one of the whole grain cold cereals, bran, wheat germ, a little plain non-fat yogurt, the best fruit of the season, and a few nuts and seeds. This is accompanied by a big pot of an herb tea, like camomile or a spice blend. It is a large breakfast, containing more than one-third of my daily calories, but it is my hungriest time of day, probably because my body has just spent so many calories in exercising.

Lunch is often just fruit—as much as I feel like eating that day—from two to four pieces. In the summer it's difficult to decide among all the beautiful selections in the produce department. In the winter, I like baked yams, baked potatoes, butternut and acorn squash, big apples, pineapple, whatever feels right that day. I actually prefer to eat lunch at home if I can.

Dinner is always vegetable time for me. Salads made with

romaine, or other dark lettuce, sometimes kale or collards shredded very fine. Then steamed or baked vegetables, potatoes, or a grain. I often add cooked brown rice right into my big salad, where the no-oil dressing makes other flavorings unnecessary. In winter I make a lot of soups, like vegetable, lentil, barley, or bean. Sometimes I buy a small piece of fish if it looks appealing at the market.

I go to sleep relatively early, so I am not troubled by food cravings in the evening. I get up VERY early in the morning, always hungry!

Beverages

Water

Water is the drink of choice. Drink large quantities of the purest water you can find in your area, preferably between meals. The additional fiber intake on a diet high in complex carbohydrates makes adequate fluid intake very important.

Studies have shown that many overweight people drink too little water. Many have told me that they don't get thirsty, and never think of getting a drink, but this is a habit pattern that can and should be changed. At first, drink a little water even when you're not thirsty, and eventually you will get used to being "hydrated."

Ironically, water is the best natural diuretic, actually counteracting any tendency toward fluid retention. Other benefits include giving a feeling of fullness, and replacing fluids lost through exercise. Many beauty experts feel that drinking plenty of water is the best technique for maintaining a glowing complexion.

Often, people confuse hunger with thirst. When your body is sending you a signal that it "wants something," but you're not absolutely sure what it is, try a big glass of water before going in search of something to eat.

If possible, keep a large glass constantly filled on your desk at work. Carry a bottle of good water in the car when the trip will be long. And it doesn't have to be kept chilled; drinking water at room temperature has one advantage—you can drink more of it.

There are now many plain or flavored varieties of sparkling waters on the market. These are delightful, and might serve as an aid in moving away from soda pop. Make sure the one you choose has no sodium.

Soft Drinks (Soda)

Soda is a non-food—the quintessential source of empty calories. Regular kinds contain up to nine teaspoons of sugar in an eight ounce serving.

The artificially sweetened varieties merely substitute man-made ingredients for the sugar; but both contain long lists of artificial colors, flavors, unpronounceable chemicals, and often caffeine.

These artifically sweetened soft drinks are a crutch for the chronic dieter. Some very fat people can be observed dropping many cans of diet soda into their shopping carts and regularly ordering them when away from home. Advertisements showing scantily clad, skinny models hold out a promise that those figures can be yours, if only you sip the same soft drink. Yet year after year, they frolic in the surf as thin as ever, while your body undergoes little, if any, change. As with any tool that has not proven useful, diet soft drinks should be discarded.

There are disturbing scientific questions about the safety of artificial sweeteners in general. Saccharin was used widely until some animals studies raised suspicions about its possible link to cancer. Now aspartame (NutraSweet and Equal) has gained wide popularity. Although its composition is more "natural" than products previously used, the Food and Drug Administration has received numerous complaints of unpleasant side effects linked to the consumption of products containing this substance.

As you are about to make one of these drinks a part of your body, read the label, and ask yourself whether the ingredients they contain have been around *long enough* for us to know their *long-range* effects. Like saccharin, many products are approved at first; it is only when new data appear that their safety is called into question.

All artificial sweeteners, in any of their forms, should be phased out of your life. That one choice is an important step toward living in a healthier, more natural way. Your long-range goal is to modify your palate so that a perfectly ripened fruit tastes satisfyingly sweet, and artificials taste cloyingly over-sweet. Many, many clients have told me that after staying away from these products for a month, they taste unpleasant and artificial. It may be difficult at first to break the soft-drink habit, but in time you will be much happier without these unnatural, non-foods in your life.

Juices

Juices have a reputation for being very good for you. While surely preferable to soda, there are reasons why they shouldn't be a big part of your diet. Juices are a fractionated food—use is made of only part of the original fruit or vegetable. Much of the fiber and many other beneficial components are discarded with the pulp.

The calorie count is relatively high for these drinks: eight ounces of orange juice is about 120 calories. You would have to squeeze between three and five oranges in order to produce eight ounces of liquid. The juice goes down quickly, and doesn't take up much room, while in the unlikely event that you ate five whole oranges at one sitting, you would be very full.

Without fiber to slow down the rate of absorption, an abrupt rising and then falling of blood sugar occurs. In this sense, the body treats the juice more like refined sugar than a whole natural food. If you are thirsty, drink water. If you really feel like having juice, try diluting it with half the amount of water.

Coffee, Tea, and Other Beverages

While everyone knows that coffee and tea contain caffeine, studies differ about how harmful this substance may be. If however, you are three or four cup a day coffee drinker who has ever given up the beverage "cold turkey," you know from experience that caffeine is indeed a drug. The withdrawal symptoms, including headache, irritability, and lethargy can be quite severe.

Some decaffeination processes are suspect, while others ("water process" or "European process") seem safe. So you have to sort out the evidence and decide whether any kind of coffee should be part of your life. Since coffee drinking is just a habit, with sufficient motivation you can phase it out of your routine if that is your choice. On the other hand, you may decide that in moderation, the pleasures of drinking regular or decaffeinated coffee and tea outweigh the potential problems unless and until new data prove otherwise.

Many people rely on caffeine to provide a needed spurt of energy. You may find, as others have, that by switching to a highly nutritious diet and following a regular exercise program, you will feel more energized and alert naturally, and no longer feel the need for the artificial stimulation of a drug.

If you do drink coffee, please avoid the use of non-dairy creamers. Reading the label on these products is a lesson in chemistry. Besides all their artificials and preservatives, they rely heavily on coconut and palm oil, two highly saturated fats. In fact, some of them contain more fat than the milk you might have used. It is true that these products contain no cholesterol, but remember, foods that have no cholesterol can still be high in fat. Switch to skimmed milk for your coffee or tea. At first, it will taste a little "thin," but like everything else, in a short time you will get used to it.

Some coffee substitutes made from cereal grains and other natural ingredients are low in calories and very good tasting. Postum and Pero are popular choices, but my favorite is Bambu, a Swiss import. It has only two calories per cup, and with a little non-fat milk, I find it to be a very satisfying hot drink.

Some herb teas are excellent (camomile, linden, orange spice) while others can taste awful. One major brand, Celestial Seasonings, offers variety packs, allowing you to sample a number of different flavors.

Don't forget clear vegetable broths are an excellent pick-me-up at any time of day or evening. Read labels for sodium content, and find those without artificial ingredients and pre-servatives. Two that I especially like are Bernard Jensen's Natu-ral Vegetable Seasoning and Instant Gravy, and Dr. Bronner's "Balanced Protein-Seasoning." Both can be found at health food stores, or can be ordered for you.

Alcohol

Alcoholic beverages have been part of human civilization since it's beginnings—as medicine, as an integral part of rites and ceremonies, as a component of festive meals. Today, con-sumption of some sort of alcoholic beverage exists in virtually every society in the world.

With the exception of some trace elements in wine, alcohol supplies only empty calories—seven per gram. Gin, scotch, vodka, etc. contain about 95–125 calories for one and a half ounces (the average drink), depending on the proof. Beer is about 150 calories for a twelve ounce glass, lite beer is under 100 calories. Wine is roughly 100 calories for a four ounce glass.

There are two important reasons to be cautious in your approach to alcohol. The first is that alcohol increases your appetite, and puts the censor in your brain to sleep—or at least renders it less effective. After a few drinks, you forget why it was so important not to have that third piece of pie. Alcohol con-sumption causes adult reason and resolve to give way to more child-like wants and desires.

Secondly, the devastating effects of overconsumption of alcohol on the body, the family, and on society are well-docu-mented and should be considered very seriously. There are people who must abstain completely. It is interesting to note, however, that some doctors continue to prescribe moderate use of alcohol to selected patients for its calming effects.

Many people consider some form of alcohol (increasing numbers are turning to wine and beer, and away from "hard liquor") as a part of the Good Life. As such, they are willing to spend the necessary calories, empty or not. If you are not a victim of alcoholism or other limiting disease, and if you like the taste of some of these beverages, the CNC Plan recognizes its moderate, temperate use. At carefully chosen times and events, alcoholic beverages can enhance and enrich one's experience and pleasure. There are some beautiful wines (make mine Champagne!) in the world, waiting to be enjoyed. Even less-than-noble vintages from the supermarket shelf can offer relaxation, enhance the taste of food, the level of conversation, and give a lift to the spirit. An ice cold beer at the ball park, a frosty gin and tonic on a warm summer evening, and a snifter of good brandy by the fire in winter may be pleasures you choose to judiciously balance into your life.

In Praise of Breakfast

Breakfast is the most important meal of the day.

Eat breakfast like a king, lunch like a prince, dinner like a pauper.

Fill the car with gas before the trip, not after you get back to the driveway.

We've heard this sort of wisdom for many years. Why, then, do so many people skip breakfast entirely, or gobble down a pastry and coffee on the run? Here are the usual reasons:

1. *Habit.* What you are used to doing or not doing tends to continue, unless you are very motivated to make a change.

2. *Eating all evening.* The typical behavior of an over-weight person is to have a large meal at the end of the day. But it is an endless meal, with snacking and nibbling continuing until bedtime. No wonder the morning is not greeted in a state of ravenous hunger. It is interesting to note that when people **DO** go to sleep after a very light evening meal, they often report feeling thin, "lean and mean," and pleasantly hungry on arising.

3. *Saving calories.* Many overweight people skip breakfast entirely, with the thought that these "saved" calories will put them ahead of the game for the rest of the day. Unfortunately, it doesn't work that way. Most people just end up eating more at

lunch and dinner, as though the body was determined to get a certain amount of food anyway, regardless of the time.

There are negative effects of the omission of breakfast that are counterproductive to weight loss and good health. The classic Iowa Breakfast Studies of 1962 as well as the research of Dr. Pollitt at the University of Texas School of Public Health, and research at the National Institutes of Health all point to reduced physical and mental performance without a morning meal (Barnett: 1986; Meer: 1986; National Institute of Health: 1981). It appears that fat is burned more efficiently in the presence of carbohydrates. Without ingested fuel, the body gears into a starvation mode, lowering the basal metabolic rate, and therefore burning calories at a *slower* rate.

4. "I'm just not hungry." Some body signals when ignored long enough, will disappear. It is likely that at some point in your life there was a desire to eat upon arising—after all, you had been "fasting" throughout the night. But if that drive has been ignored for a long time, the thought of eating early in the day may not be pleasant. These dormant signals can be reawakened, and a new pattern of morning hunger can be established over time.

5. "There's not enough time in the morning—I'm too rushed." If taking care of the body is high on one's list of priorities, then planning and providing necessary body fuel for a productive day must take precedence over a few extra minutes of sleep. The act of preparing just the right breakfast, and making time to enjoy it (perhaps with the morning paper) is symbolic of a healthy self concern. All mothers are famous for urging you to eat a good breakfast. Now be your own good mother, and take the best care of yourself.

Many overweight people eat only one meal a day. Few normal weight people follow this practice. Here are some strategies for establishing a routine of breakfast eating:

- Limit or discontinue nighttime snacking. Picture your digestive system as closed and locked after the evening meal, not to reopen until breakfast.

- Get up a little earlier. The morning is a perfect time to exercise, and the activity will increase your appetite.

- Start with a small piece of fruit. In time, you will find some whole grain cereal or a muffin sounds appealing.

- Pack a brown bag of nutritious foods to be eaten when hunger appears. Since this is impossible for school children, it is even more important for a healthy pattern of breakfast eating to be established in the household.

It is unfair to yourself to try and face the world without the protection of a full stomach and a stable blood sugar level. No one should have to resist a cart of sweet pastries at 11:00 A.M. on an empty stomach. They will always **look good to you,** but after your nourishing breakfast, you are much more likely to decide to pass them up.

Calorie Bargains

Here are some calorie bargains that give lots of taste and/or fun value at very little calorie cost:

Mustard. Whether it's old-fashioned yellow, spicy brown or the exotic and expensive Dijon and other European varieties, it has only 15 calories per tablespoon, yet imparts a lot of flavor, and seems so "creamy." Compare it to another sandwich spread, mayonnaise, weighing in at 100 calories per tablesoon.

Parmesan Cheese. When it is grated, this delicious food is mostly air. Therefore for about twenty-five calories per tablespoon, you can get a real Italian taste.

Air-popped popcorn. At twenty-three calories per cup (with no butter or oil, you can keep chewing this fun-food until your jaws get tired, with the added bonus that it's high in fiber and very nutritious.

Soup. Mostly any kind except "creamed" supplies few calories, but makes you feel very full and satisfied.

Foods that take a long time to eat. Enjoy an artichoke (slowly!) dipped in a non-fat dressing. Munch a large apple, savoring each bite. All this chewing gives the satiety center in your brain time to register fullness. Since high-fiber foods take longer to chew, eating them may help you slow down your eating.

Mexican-style Salsa (without oil), adds spice to many foods, and is a good way to move away from fatty condiments. Try it on a baked potato, or a warmed (not fried) corn or flour tortilla, heaped with shredded lettuce and cooked (no oil) beans.

Make creamy, rich tasting toppings by whipping canned *evaporated skimmed milk*.

Sun-Dried Tomatoes. The darlings of nouvelle cuisine, are now available in cellophane packages, with no preservatives, and no oil. They add a lot of flavor and panache to salads and many other foods. Like all dried fruits, use them sparingly, because you could quite easily eat the equivalent of three or four fresh tomatoes at one time, which could add up to roughly 120 calories.

Vinegars. Many fancy vinegars are in the markets—some with herbs floating in the bottles. Rice vinegar is very mellow, and some people find it the best to use if you're avoiding any oil. All vinegars are virtually calorie-free.

Baked vegetables. Try almost any vegetables baked in a hot oven or microwave until they are barely tender. Eggplant, bell peppers, Brussels sprouts, and especially mushrooms taste amazingly good this way without the addition of any sauce or fat. Or, bake a whole, unpeeled, yellow onion until it is quite soft. Then peel and eat. It will have lost its "bite," and taste very sweet. Of course it is extremely low in calories.

Helpful Hints for Your New Style of Eating

▶ Shop for fresh produce as often as possible. Plan your meals around the most beautiful fruits and vegetables available each day. A great chef was asked what he was preparing for dinner that evening. "How can I say?" he replied, "I haven't yet been to the market."

▶ Read every label of every food that goes into your body. If you can't pronounce it, don't eat it. If it comes in a box, package, or can, it's probably not as good for you as a whole, living food. Usually, with packaged foods, the more complicated the ingredient list, the more fat and calories they contain.

Labels list ingredients in the order of their relative weight in the product. The most prominent ingredient is listed first, and so on. For example, beware of a box of cereal that lists sugar and/ or dextrose, corn syrup, or any sweetener first. You will be eating a lot of empty calories and not enough of the grain shown on the box to make it a good nutritional value.

The labels of some products on the market list *no real food at all!* They read like a witch's brew of chemicals, artificials, and preservatives (For example, check the artificial whipped cream). Reading a few of these can help propel you toward a more natural way of eating. Plan for your trips to the store to take longer at first, because reading labels takes time. (Isn't it interesting that fruits, vegetables, grains and legumes don't need any labels?)

▶ Even though you can find almost everything you need in a regular market, it's a good idea to locate a "health food" or "natural food" store in your neighborhood. It will become a valuable source of whole foods, many packaged with no pre-servatives or artificial ingredients. Walk up and down the aisles, discovering items that are new to you, and don't hesitate to ask employees for help. Be careful! Just because you find a food in a health food store doesn't mean it's automatically low calorie or superior nutritionally—keep reading labels. Many of these stores also have book departments which feature recipes for cooking natural foods.

▶ Plan a lot of meals around soup. Clear broths are useful before, between, or with meals, while main-dish soups provide the opportunity to use legumes, vegetables and grains in deli-cious, satisfying combinations. Both are great helps in making you feel full and satisfied. People who eat a lot of soup have described it as very useful in weight loss.

To thicken soup, purée some or all of the beans or vegeta-bles after they are cooked. Flavor with broth or seasonings (see page **58** for suggestions), then cook rice, barley, or other grains directly in this rich "stock." At the last minute, add more vegetables to be cooked *al dente* (firm). You have created a very satisfying and nutritious one-dish meal.

▶ Whip mashed potatoes with non-fat milk instead of butter, cream, or whole milk. Then add flavor with herbs, spices, or a pinch of powdered vegetable broth. They are fluffy and delicious, and certainly don't make you feel you are "on a diet."

▶ Buy an air popper. Air-popped popcorn (without butter or oil) is a low calorie (twenty-three per cup), nutritious, high-fiber snack. Best of all, it's fun, doesn't bear the stigma of a "diet food," and takes a long time to eat! I wish we could get this kind of popcorn at the movies, but even without adding that optional squirt of butter, it still seems to be popped in some kind of fat. As yet I've been unable to find a brand of popcorn packaged for microwaves that is fat-free, but I'm sure it's only a matter of time before one appears on the market.)

▶ Baked potatoes, lobster, green vegetables, and corn on the cob are just some of the foods with delicious flavors that can stand alone. Slathering them with butter masks their natural tastes. Eat them on their own for a month, and you won't miss the old, high-calorie way.

▶ The foods of affluence—high-fat marbled meats, rich cheeses, creamy creations, fancy pastries, highly refined white flour and sugar, have brought with them the *diseases* of affluence. Eat like a peasant! Coarse-grain breads, thick homemade soups, fresh seasonal fruits and vegetables make you healthier, slimmer, and leave you with more money in your pocket at the end of the week. The more processed the food, usually the more it costs. Frozen dinners, boxes of cookies, and canned meats are much more expensive than a bag of beans, a pound of rice, and a sack of potatoes.

▶ Since fat has nine calories per gram, and protein and carbohydrates have four calories per gram, surprising as it may seem, you are better off "splurging" on a sugary food than on a fatty one, like a cheeseburger or French fries.

Although fats and sugar usually go together, there are some sweets with a relatively low fat content. Sometimes, just allowing yourself one or two hard candies can ward off an impending high-fat, high calorie binge. Here are some no-fat or very low fat sweet foods:

angel food cake	frozen fruit bars
sponge cake	hard candy, jelly beans
water ices	meringues
"sugar" cookies	fig bars
ginger snaps	animal crackers

▶ Explore all herbs and spices, both dried and fresh. Try Veg-it or Lawry's Natural Choice as substitutes for salt. Lemon juice is a helpful seasoning on vegetables and fish. There are fruit concentrates that come frozen (apple juice is especially useful) or in little bottles that look like syrups, that are good sweetners. Or make your own sweetener by puréeing very ripe fruit in a blender or processor (try strawberries or raspberries). These pure flavors will help you get used to a more natural sweet taste.

▶ There are many new products (the list grows every day) that are low in calories, but **do not rely on artificial sweeteners or flavorings.** In your desire to be slim, don't fall victim to the practice of eating "chemical foods" in order to save calories.

You can now buy jams and jellies made only with fruit, without sugar or artificials of any kind, containing very few calories per teaspoon; many new frozen desserts are naturally sweetened; many brands of cold cereals are free of artificial colorings or flavorings, and taste delicious.

Keep looking for and buying these healthier items. Manufacturers will be encouraged to take a more natural approach if that's what the public wants.

▶ You can make or buy low-calorie Marinara-style tomato sauces for pasta that contain no oil or sugar. Then add onions, garlic, eggplant, mushrooms, zucchini, etc. directly to the bubbling sauce, instead of sautéeing the vegetables first in fat.

▶ All complex carbohydrates are relatively low in calories because of their high water and/or fiber content, and low fat percentages. From lowest to highest calorie count they are:

vegetables   fruits   grains   legumes

▶ Cook with a new freedom. Just as this program doesn't offer a rigid, strict diet for you to follow, you are encouraged to be free and creative as you explore the world of fresh, natural foods. Modify and invent recipes as the spirit moves you. If the recipe calls for rice, and you feel like barley, go for it!

▶ Food preparation in this more natural eating style may take a bit longer (rinsing or peeling fruits and vegetables; making your own soups), but you make up for it at clean-up time. Greasy meat pans are harder to scrub than salad bowls.

▶ Nutritional yeast (brewer's yeast) has been claimed by some to be an energy-giving wonder food. It does have some strong points—for about twenty-three calories a tablespoon, you get a generous dose of B vitamins, plus a high percentage of fat-free protein.

Its major drawback has been a less-than-wonderful flavor, but advances have been made. Now, there are some brands on the market that are quite tasty when sprinkled on salads, cereals, in juices, or blender "health" drinks. I like it in soups to add extra richness, but my favorite way is to sprinkle it over just-cooked brown rice. One good-tasting brand you mighty try is KAL.

▶ When selecting fruit, pick the heaviest specimen of its kind. It is the one which usually has the most juice (pineapple, grapefruit, orange, melon).

▶ Try these frozen fruit treats: peel a fully ripe banana (yellow, and flecked with brown "sugar spots"), wrap it in aluminum foil or plastic wrap, and freeze. Eat it like a popsickle when it is frozen solid, or whirl it in the food processor or blender. Its consistency will resemble that of vanilla ice cream. Add a bit of cinnamon or vanilla if you like, spoon it into the center of a halved canteloupe, or add pited cherries for a low-calorie "cherry vanilla" delight.

Grapes, taken off the stem, and blueberries, popped into freezer bags become like hard little candies, fun to suck on, and very sweet tasting. Because they take a long time to eat, you will find yourself eating smaller quantities.

▶ If a high complex-carbohydrate diet is new to you, make the switch slowly. Both your habit patterns and your digestive system need time to get used to the change. Gradually increase the proportion of darker greens in the salad; switch from whole milk to low-fat, then eventually to non-fat; make your portions of animal protein smaller and smaller; increase the size of your salad every day.

▶ When I first started to cook brown rice according to standard directions (2 cups of water to 1 cup of rice), it always came out mushy and soft. I evolved my own unorthodox technique that I'd like to share with you. I hope it helps, because brown rice is one of the most nutritious, staple foods you can eat.

Bring about one cup of water to a boil. Lightly rinse about ⅔ cup rice in a strainer, then add it to the boiling water. When it returns to a boil, stir, and skim off the "stuff" that comes to the surface. The rice should be covered by no more than one-half inch of water at this point. Cover the pot, and simmer until all the water is absorbed. Taste the rice for chewiness as you go. You want it to be firm, but not too hard. You can always add a little extra water while it's cooking, but once it's mushy from too much liquid, there's nothing you can do. Be careful to see that the bottom of the pot doesn't burn. Each kernel of rice should come out firm and separate, and ready to flavor in any way you choose.

▶ After a time of "festive" eating, many of my clients have enjoyed a day or more of eating only raw foods—fruits, vegetables and sprouts. It is a very low-calorie way to eat, and gives the feeling of "cleansing" the body.

▶ Notice the colors of the food in your shopping cart and on your plate. Fresh fruits and vegetables are vibrant with bright color (when not overcooked), while meats, gravies, and many processed foods tend to be dull.

▶ Here's a tip for taking good care of yourself: If you have an emotional issue to discuss with someone, the **LAST** place you should do it is over a meal. Digestion is impeded by strong emotional responses, and you should never eat when you are upset. Heavy issues should always be discussed in a non-food environment.

▶ If you want to keep your calories very low, but you're not quite full after a meal, "top off your tank" with a warm drink. Broth, herb tea, or coffee substitutes are very good for this purpose.

▶ You don't have to put your barbeque away if you decide to eat less red meat. Of course chicken works beautifully, as does any firm-fleshed fish, like salmon, halibut, swordfish or shrimp. Here's something new to try: leave young vegetables whole, or cut almost any vegetable up into chunks. Cook them over charcoal or the new fragrant wood chips, and you'll find they take on a delicious flavor.

▶ When you're not quite sure if you're really hungry, a good rule is:

WHEN IN DOUBT, DO WITHOUT.

When you're not quite sure whether you feel like exercising, the rule is:

WHEN IN DOUBT, DO!

▶ No one is sure why this trick works so well, but it does: When you have eaten all you have planned for a particular meal (especially in the evening), go and thoroughly brush your teeth. The taste of the toothpaste, or the ritual itself tells the body that eating is over for now. Many have used this strategy to break the habit pattern of eating continuously from dinner to bedtime.

▶ Start each meal with the lowest calorie items. For example, cut-up raw vegetables first, then a big green salad, then a cup of vegetable broth would leave you little room for anything else. You will be very full on very few calories.

▶ Clean out your kitchen! Developing strong will-power is not your goal; making life easy for yourself is. Sure you can drive down to the store at any time to buy cookies, but you are less likely to do so than you are to tiptoe to the kitchen at night to forage for what's already there. Ask for the cooperation of those you live with. If you don't want a certain food around because it has a lot of fat and calories, it's probably better for everyone to banish it from your home.

If there are children in your household it is even more important to be nutritionally aware. Their young bodies are being built every day with the raw materials you buy and prepare. Take a stand! If they (and you) eat in a healthy manner at home, the "damage" done by junk food in the outside world is much less significant in terms of overall health.

Vitamin and Mineral Supplements

Vitamins and minerals are absolutely essential for life and health. They are found in the foods we eat and the pills we may choose to buy.

Should you supplement your diet with vitamins and minerals, and if so, in what dosages? Is one kind of vitamin more "natural" or effective than another?

Of all the controversial issues in the field of nutrition, this subject seems the most puzzling. "Expert" advice ranges from many medical doctors who assure us that just by eating a "balanced diet" (whatever that means), our nutrient needs will be met, to Linus Pauling's well-known recommendations for megadoses of vitamin C (Pauling: 1970).

Here are some well known theories for supplementing our diets with vitamins and minerals:

• Our soils have been depleted so that the foods we grow may be lacking in some important nutrients.
• The effects of environmental pollutants on our bodies can be counteracted by taking certain supplements.
• Because of our hectic life-styles, we often don't eat the way we should.
• Over-processed foods are stripped of the nutritive value with which they were originaly endowed.
• Certain medications and practices (cigarette smoking, alcohol and sugar comsumption), along with stress deplete our stores of some vitamins (the B complex and C).

• Some diseases might be prevented or lessened through mineral supplementation (calcium for osteoporosis).
• Pregnancy and old-age may create increased needs for specific nutrients.

On the other side of the argument, a compelling case can be made for spending your money on a wide variety of nutritious food, instead of on expensive pills.

I'm not going to offer direct advice about whether you should take supplements or not, because the evidence doesn't seem conclusive either way. I do want to give you some guidelines that might help you make your own decisions:

• Read and listen to the opinions of a variety of experts. Pay attention to the scientific data backing up their opinions.
• Tune in to any reactions you can sense in your own body when you do take supplements. (Do you avoid or lessen a cold after taking large amounts of vitamin C?)
• Don't take high dosages ("megadoses") of anything without serious research and consultation with a reliable authority.
• Keep an open mind and be flexible. Watch for today's accepted practice to become tomorrow's discarded theory.
• Most important, if you take vitamin pills, don't develop a false sense of security. Supplements do not substitute for healthy eating, but are merely an adjunct to it.

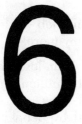

Choosing
Exercise

▶ **BE SURE TO CHECK WITH YOUR PHYSICIAN
BEFORE YOU EMBARK ON ANY EXERCISE PROGRAM.**

The Usual Excuses

How often have you heard (or used) one of the following excuses for not exercising?

"I'm just too busy. There's no way I could fit it in. If you knew what my day was like, you'd understand."

"I'm really lazy. I hate exercise. It's for jocks, not me. Some people just aren't cut out for it."

"Whenever I work out, I just get hungrier, so what's the point?

"Once I followed an exercise program for a while and all I did was gain weight."

"I'm not going to a gym with all those thin people. I'm embarrassed to be seen in a leotard or shorts."

"I would exercise, but it makes me perspire. My mother always told me that was unhealthy. Besides, it ruins my make-up."

"It's too hot. Nobody can even move in this humidity, much less exercise."

"I get plenty of exercise walking around on my job (or lifting boxes, or chasing kids). So I don't need to do any more."

"Maybe other people have to sweat and suffer. I can lose weight by just cutting down on what I eat. I've done it a million times." (!?!)

Throw out these excuses! They are used by people who have not been successful in controlling their weight permanently. As you read this chapter, I hope you decide that you no longer need excuses, and begin to see why exercise **MUST** be part of your life.

The Pleasure of Eating More

The most compelling reason to exercise can be illustrated by relating a casual conversation I overheard one day while pedaling along on the exercise bicycle at my gym. Next to me was a slim, good-looking man with a reputation for being a "party animal." A friend of his walked by, playfully rifling the pages of the newspaper he was reading. "Hey Bill," he said, "you really work hard at this, don't you!" "You bet," said Bill, grinning and wiping the perspiration from his face. "This is the hard part of the good life."

That little scene sums up the philosophy of the Choosing Not Cheating Plan. Nothing is free. Everything has its cost. A price must be paid so that eating can be a pleasure of life instead of a source of varying degrees of anguish. A major part of that price is making the effort and taking the time to build a lean body that will be on your side, ready to burn calories effectively through exercise. As difficult as it might seem at first,

IT IS MUCH EASIER TO EXERCISE MORE
THAN IT IS TO EAT LESS.

The slim, handsome actor Bruce Dern was heard to say on a talk show that he is an avid jogger not so much because he loves to run, but because he loves to eat.

Our Animal Selves

In *The White Peacock* D. H. Lawrence said, "Be a good animal, true to your animal instincts." These words are worth remembering when the demands and pressures of modern life cause us to lose touch with our animal selves. Our bodies were equipped with large muscles in the legs and buttocks so we could forage, compete with other animals for food, and flee an attacking predator. Clearly this musculature was not created for spending eight hours behind a desk. If you're like most people, when you think through your day you will be amazed at just how sedentary you've become. The typical path goes from bed to car to desk to car to couch, and back to bed.

Humans today tend to be more intellectual than physical. They ignore or neglect the body, while emphasizing and relying on what goes on in the head. If you picture a person suited to this sort of existence, it would be a science-fiction character with a huge head and a tiny, atrophied body. But no matter how far civilization has advanced, the body's muscular structure has remained the same, and needs to be used. Not exercising your body is like keeping a thoroughbred horse locked in the barn, never allowing it to run free.

The "fight or flight" mechanism that prepared us to repel or escape from a wild animal is still very much with us. Even though today's stressor might be the boss rather than a sabre-toothed tiger, the most effective, healthiest reaction to tension is still to release it through movement.

We are paying a high price for becoming "advanced" and freed from physical labor. We suffer from degenerative diseases in epidemic proportions, many caused or made worse by obesity. The U.S. Department of Health and Human Services says that thirty-two million Americans are overweight, and that this condition is primarily the result of very low levels of physical activity, rather than excess consumption of calories.

When lean rats are caged, they become overweight even when their diet remains constant. When **WE** don't *move* enough, the beautiful human body that was designed to be of normal weight, usually becomes fat and out of shape.

We know that a moving body demands more energy (calories) than a body at rest. When constant movement was a necessary part of daily life, we needed a lot of food for fuel. Now we still want the food but thanks to our modern conveniences, our bodies actually move around much less and, therefore, burn fewer calories.

Cavemen didn't need to lift weights at the gym—they lifted real boulders. In fact, up until very modern times, physical labor was a part of everyone's life. Now, we have to restore the physical activity that modern civilization has taken away.

Ed McMahon once joked on television, "I don't have to exercise, I get someone else to do it for me." As much as some people might wish that were possible, exercise is one of the few activities that you must do yourself.

Sedentary people have also lost some other things of value: the joy of body movement; the exhilaration and feeling of well-being that comes from strenuous physical activity; the child-like delight in play.

The "Magic Bullet"

What if I told you there really **was** a cure for overweight—a "magic bullet" that would end the problem forever. You'd probably be willing to pay any price, or travel anywhere to find it. The irony is that the solution is simple and within your reach. All the research now shows that exercising the right way on a consistent basis is *the key* to a lifetime of successful weight management.

If you are overweight, and decide to make no changes in your eating pattern, but start doing a reasonable amount of correct exercise, you **will** lose weight. Guaranteed. If you combine the exercise with proper eating, the ball game is over, and you are the winner. Exercise is so vital, that as surprising as it may seem, if I were forced to choose between adherence to a low-fat diet, or to an excellent exercise plan, I would have to choose the latter. Exercise is at least 50% of losing weight and more important, of keeping it off.

Why Is Exercise So Important?

When you try to take off pounds by following a low-calorie diet without exercise, the body senses impending starvation and

lowers the rate at which calories are burned. Weakness and hunger make you feel fatigued, so you move around less, thus conserving even more fat. The result is that all your valiant efforts are counterproductive. The more will power you muster and the less you eat, the more your own body sabatoges the effort, tenaciously holding on to its fat stores.

Authorities don't agree on specific numbers, but the normal percentage of body fat for men is about 10–15%, and for women 18–25%. Anything above these numbers is unattractive and unhealthy, and it is this extra fat that should be the target of a weight reduction program. But most people give no thought to WHAT they are "losing" when they "go on a diet." All they want to do is lose weight.

On the typical very low-calorie diet or fast, a lot of weight is lost quickly, but that weight is composed of water and muscle as well as fat. This loss of lean body mass is counterproductive, because *the only way to get rid of fat is to burn it in the muscles.* You need all the muscle tissue you can get!

An arm or leg that was just removed from a cast has lost its tone and looks shrunken and withered from being immobile. It is only by exercising correctly that you actually preserve and increase your muscle mass—in effect creating little fat-burning factories to work for you. The bonus is that the accelerated rate of calorie burning produced by exercising continues not only while you're engaged in the activity, but remains revved up long after, even when you're asleep. Exercise thus has benefits that go beyond the calories burned while you're working out. Your body becomes more efficient at burning calories while at rest, and less efficient at storing them for the remainder of the day. In fact, the actual number of calories burned during exercise is quite small—a 150-pound person burns only about 100 calories per mile of walking—equal to the calories in one good-sized apple. The change in metabolism brought about by exercise is the important factor.

Fat cells are inert. They don't need any fuel. But muscles demand energy. So the more lean muscle mass, the greater the energy requirement and the more calories are burned. When you have reduced your percentage of muscle cells through repeated dieting, you no longer use up fat as well as someone who has never dieted at all. Because each time you "gain all the weight back," it's not regained in the same proportions—you get back *less* muscle and *more* fat. In fact, if you had never gotten on the diet merry-go-round and you reduced your percentage of lean muscle tissue, you might be slightly overweight today, but probably not obese.

Linda, a psychotherapist, had been on many diets over the years, but had never understood the exercise component of weight reduction. She had lost and gained literally hundreds of pounds and was still left with a very high percentage of body fat. My first task was to convince her that exercise was 50% of our **permanent** weight-loss plan. She reluctantly agreed to give it a try.

I had recommended that she weigh herself only once a month, but the next week she confessed that she didn't feel like she was losing much, so she got on the scale to see "how much less I have to eat to lose weight." She was so conditioned to eliminating more and more food to achieve weight loss (always temporary), she didn't know the right question would have been, "How much more do I have to excercise to lose fat?" Eventually, she became convinced that the benefit of being able to eat more on a regular basis and not restrict herself so rigidly all the time (between times of bingeing) was reason enough to stick to the exercise program.

Always trying to cut back on your food intake to get slim becomes increasingly difficult as time goes on. Each year, as the metabolic rate slows down with aging you have to eat less to maintain the same weight. Depriving yourself, relying on will power, constantly thinking about food because you're just a little hungry is a painful, unnatural thing to do.

But here's the good news: as you increase the proportion of muscle tissue in your body, you get to eat more, since it takes more calories to maintain muscle than fat. Two women may both weigh 130 pounds on the scale, but if one has a low percentage of body fat and a high percentage of muscle, she can *eat more* to maintain the *same weight* than another woman with more fat and less muscle.

Thus by increasing your body's percentage of lean muscle tissue, you can eat and enjoy food more. That is an important, achievable result of the CNC Plan. But be prepared: muscle tissue weights more than fat. As you increase the proportion of muscle to fat, your scale weight could actually go up temporarily.

An uninformed, battle-scarred dieter could hastily decide that this plan isn't working, when in reality it's working perfectly.

Although the scale may show little or no reduction in the beginning, your body will definitely be changing and your clothes fitting in a different way. Exercised muscles elongate, getting slimmer and shaplier, and a leaner, firmer body begins to emerge. These signs are the true measures of your success.

You will be very aware now when you hear people discussing "weight" loss, that the critical measure should be "fat" loss. The best question one could ask a person who is trying to get slim is, "How much muscle tissue have you built?"

Of course you will see a reduction in scale weight but— with a difference. On crash diets, you lose the most in the beginning, then hit the infamous plateau. By eating a diet high in complex carbohydrates and low in fat, never "starving yourself" on less than 1,200 calories a day, and increasing your physical activity, the rate of loss is likely to go **UP** over time, as you build more fat-burning muscle cells.

More Benefits of Exercise

For the purpose of weight control, one of the biggest advantages of exercise is that it helps to reduce your appetite. But be forewarned: when a very overweight individual *begins* an exercise program, the appetite will probably *increase* **temporarily**. This happens because obese people don't burn fat efficiently. The increase in activity causes blood glucose to be used for fuel, which stimulates hunger. However, with a continued program of regular exercise, the body will begin to mobilize its *fat stores* for energy, and an exercise session will depress rather than increase the appetite.

Below are some additional, extremely positive benefits of exercise.

• *The heart is strengthened.* Because the heart is a muscle, exercise increases its efficiency, making it bigger and stronger. The pulse rate decreases—it doesn't have to work as hard to pump blood through the body—and the risk of heart attack is reduced. Some people have called the legs auxiliary pumps for the heart.

• *Blood pressure is lowered.* Improved blood circulation increases the amount of oxygen to all the cells. You feel energized, don't get tired or out of breath as easily, and you see your complexion and skin-tone improve. Blood pressure is lowered, and so is the risk of getting a stroke. Regular exercise increases HDL cholesterol—the protective "good" kind—which has been linked to decreased risk of coronary artery disease.

• *Life span is increased.* In a study monitoring 17,000 Harvard alumni, Dr. Ralph Paffenbarger found that individuals who walked briskly for forty-five minutes every day, or ran or swam for thirty minutes daily, had a death rate one-quarter to one-third lower than those who were sedentary. The active group lived about two years longer than the non-exercisers (Brody: 1986).

• *Tension is relieved.* Physical activity not only conditions the body, but results in improved mental health as well. Exercise has proven to be the single most effective tension reliever—a socially accepted outlet for frustration, anger, and aggressive feelings. In tests at the University of Kansas with depressed people, McCann and Holmes found exercise to be equal or better than psychotherapy in reliveing symptoms of depression (and at a fraction of the cost).

• *Achieve a natural high.* Vigorous levels of exercise release brain chemicals call endorphins, producing the feeling of being "high" without drugs. In fact, people who achieve this natural high are probably less likely to seek the artifically induced state (Brody: 1986).

• *Relieve/delay the symptoms of aging.* New, exciting research is indicating that what we have come to consider the inevitable conditions of aging are often caused by neglect or lack of the proper use of the body (Ward: 1984). By following a regular exercise routine and eating intelligently, we might be able to avoid or at least delay many of these symptoms. For example, bones are strengthened by weight-bearing exercises, and the likelihood of becoming a victim of osteoporosis, the brittle-bone syndrome, decreases. Activity keeps the joints lubricated, so they don't "creak" when we move. The skin also stays resilient longer, postponing the "crepy" look of old age.

Some scientists are postulating that animals (and perhaps people) who are very lean and trim have a better chance for longevity. Certainly we have all seen some extremely fit, youthful looking people well over the age of fifty or sixty who bear no resemblance to what stereotypical "old age" is supposed to look like.

• *Enjoy better sex.* It's worth remembering too, that sex is a physical activity. It is likely that a well-toned, fit, lean body will derive more pleasure from sexual activity than one that is out of shape. Besides, it's hard to be uninhibited when you are uncomfortable about how you look without clothes on.

• *Just for pleasure.* Speaking of pleasure, people who have become addicted to exercise will tell you that they continue not just because it keeps them in condition or allows them to eat more. It is a joyful activity in and of itself. Not all the time, not every day, but when things are right, that wonderful feeling of a healthy body moving through space more than makes up for the effort expended. Other people notice the glow of well-being that radiates from someone who has exercised vigorously.

Penance?

While I personally believe that exercise is a happy part of life, and certainly not in any way to be considered a punishment, some clients have used it effectively in that way.

If you awaken one morning feeling disgusted with yourself for some overindulgence the night before, pay your "penance" by increasing your exercise. As the going gets tough, make the connection between what you ate and the need to "pay the piper" to keep your life in balance. This is the time to ask yourself if what you ate was really worth it. Would you choose to spend *that* many calories on *that* particular food next time?

Let yourself feel "cleansed" by the physical activity. Having learned what you could from the episode, you should be ready to put it behind you.

I'm Sold on Exercise. What Next?

To achieve the goal of lifetime fitness, mount your attack from two directions: make a non-negotiable commitment to a preplanned exercise routine, and decide to add more movement to your life in every way you can.

Get Moving!

The basal metabolic rate, the rate at which your body uses calories for energy, is determined when you are at rest, performing only normal internal functions, i.e. breathing, digesting, thinking. Any increase in that baseline activity level is a positive step toward fitness. Begin to increase movement in small ways like standing instead of sitting, taking the stairs instead of the elevator, dancing around the room when a good song comes on the radio, tightening the abdominal muscles while waiting in a check-out line, carrying the golf bag instead of riding in a cart. Each of these behaviors may seem insignificant by itself, but they contribute to an over-all increase in energy (calorie) expenditure. It might be helpful to keep thinking that anytime you burn extra calories, you get to enjoy more food.

Many studies have shown that overweight people do not necessarily eat more than normal-weight people. But they consistently **move less.** In fact, they are often most inventive in finding ways to stay still and not exert themselves.

To avoid bending, some people become adept at picking things up off the floor with curled toes. Napping is a favorite sport. Even when they get themselves to a health club, they develop a great affinity for the more passive activities, like strapping a vibrating belt around the hips, and exercise that demands only that the participant stand still.

The habit of avoiding movement seems to develop early in life. If you observe a group of children at recess, it is the skinny, wiry ones who are fidgeting, wiggling, and staying in constant motion, while the overweight children find ways to avoid exertion. One child told me she brought a book to the outfield when she was forced to play softball.

Whether these differences are genetically induced, influenced by sedentary family life-styles, or caused by lack of proficiency in sports doesn't matter. It is only important to recognize that while the patterns are difficult to overcome, slowly, patiently, and with very small steps, **IT CAN BE DONE.**

Start taking stairs instead of elevators.

Walk instead of using the car or bus when possible.

Stride along the beach instead of lying on a blanket.

Volunteer to do the errand that requires a trip upstairs.

The Planned Exercise Program

There are three basic components of a comprehensive exercise program: cardiovascular conditioning, muscular strength, and flexibility.

Cardiovascular Conditioning

Cardiovacular conditioning is achieved through **aerobic** activity—which means literally to exercise with air. It is the kind of exercise that strengthens the heart, lungs, and circulatory system and promotes well-being. **It is the only kind of exercise that burns fat.**

Muscular Strength

Muscular strength is the development of strong, firm, well-shaped muscles that look great, and become your little fat burning factories. You will feel more attractive and powerful. No man or woman wants to be a wimp!

Flexibility

Flexibility is necessary to keep joints "oiled," and to maintain a supple, lithe, youthful appearance.

Cardiovascular/Aerobic Exercise

Aerobic exercise is the cornerstone of any exercise program because in addition to strengthening the cardiovascular system, it burns fat while preserving and increasing lean body mass. It is defined as non-stop, steady, rhythmic activity performed with enough energy output to increase the heart and breathing rates. The key is that the activity must continue in an uninterrupted manner for a period of twenty–thirty minutes, with the *duration* of the exercise more important than the intensity. So it would be better to ride an exercise bicycle at a lower rate for thirty minutes, than to pedal furiously for ten minutes.

The goal is to keep the heart rate in the "target zone." That means you are working hard enough to get the benefits of the activity, but not over-taxing your body. For a very overweight or out-of-shape person, working hard could mean walking half a block. For an athlete in prime condition, working hard might require a sprint to reach the proper level.

The formula for accurately finding your training heart rate is this: subtract your age from 220, which is the "standard" maximum heart rate to find **your** maximum heart rate. Then take a percentage of that number to figure out your target heart rate. That percentage varies from 60% to 85%, 60% if you're really out of shape, 85% if you're a trained athlete. Aim for 75% when you're well into your exercise program. (Bailey: 1977 and Fonda: 1984).

While you're exercising (if you can), or immediately afterward, take your pulse for ten seconds. Multiply that number by six to get a one minute pulse rate. Tailor your activity so that this number is in your target zone.

The unscientific but reliable way to determine your activity level is to look for two signs: you have begun to perspire, and, although you are breathing a bit heavily, you can still carry on a normal conversation. If it's difficult for you to talk, you are doing too much.

Some of the activities that meet these requirements are: walking, jogging, swimming, bicycling (stationary and motion), rope-jumping, rowing, cross-country skiing, ice or roller skating, or bouncing on a mini-trampoline. There are sports which appear to use a lot of energy, but do not qualify as an aerobic exercise because of frequent interruptions—too much time is spent just standing around. Baseball, bowling, and golf are some of these.

Remember, to qualify as an aerobic exercise, the activity you choose must be sustained—done for twenty to thirty minutes without interruption, brisk enough to reach your target heart rate, and done regularly, from three to six times per week.

Choosing What Works for You

Walking

The first thing to consider, especially if you've been sedentary for a while, is walking. This underrated activity is actually one of the best forms of exercise. It is free, can be done almost anytime, anywhere, has virtually no risk of injury (Choose your route carefully.) and can be modified to suit any level of fitness—even to the level of "race walking," a sport that is gaining in popularity. Walking up gentle or steep hills adds to the cardiovascular benefits of this activity.

Brisk walking on a regular basis carries with it additional health benefits like lowering blood pressure, and increasing stamina, energy, and muscle tone.

In the beginning, one block may seem difficult. Later, you may be walking many miles at a brisk pace. The only consideration to keep in mind is that you will have to walk longer and for greater distances to achieve the same level of fitness than you would get from a more strenuous workout. But so what? The activity is so pleasant that you won't be in a hurry to "get it over with."

You need no special equipment, except an excellent pair of shoes. Do not try to save money on this purchase! Go to one of the athletic stores that specialize in running and walking shoes, and try on many different brands. Don't buy anything until you find a pair that feels so good you hate to take them off. There is no such thing as a break-in period for these shoes—they must be comfortable right from the start. Keep trying on shoes until you find the model that suits you best.

Walking sessions are the perfect time to awaken a new body-awareness. Think about your posture, and what kind of image you present to someone observing you. Suck in the abdominals, tuck in the butt, pull your shoulders back, and take long strides. Walk like a positive, powerful, lean person who can set goals and achieve them.

Walking alone offers the opportunity to turn inward and think reflective thoughts, to study the natural scenery, or the changing cityscape. Many people today are wearing earphones attached to portable radios and getting lost in their own world of music or talk. A word of caution—watch out for traffic.

Walking with someone else offers different pleasures. For some reason, it seems easier to communicate at these times and affords the opportunity to discuss meaningful and emotionally-charged issues. Invite someone close to you to share a walk and enjoy both the physical benefits and the added bonus of getting closer to another person.

On Sunday mornings, my husband and I go for a very long walk. For about an hour we get to talk about things that just don't come up, or that time hasn't allowed for during the week. Sometimes a sticky issue will occur to one of us, and we say, "Let's save that one for the walk."

Running/Jogging

Running or jogging (usually defined as a slower run) is always an option. Its popularity seems to have peaked, but those who do it regularly sometimes become fanatical and wouldn't consider giving it up. The problem is that it's hard to find a runner who doesn't have a bad knee, a foot injury, shin splits, or one of an assortment of other complaints. But when everything is right, there *is* such a thing as a runner's high coming from the release of endorphins, and you develop a general feeling of well-being that lasts all day. There's no question that it's an excellent route to cardiovascular fitness. It is also free, and usually convenient. My warning about shoes is even more important if you decide to take up this sport. (Purchase the best *running shoes* available.)

Aerobic Dancing

One of the most popular ways to get a cardiovascular workout is an aerobic dancing class. To qualify, the class must include a period where the jogging or kicking does not stop for a minimum of twenty minutes. The pulsating, loud music, and the "dancing" aspects of these classes make them fun, and any activity that is fun tends to be continued. The movements are varied, and the arms and trunk are exercised as well as the large muscles of the legs and hips.

There are some dangers to watch out for. Cement floors are very hard on the body, even if they are covered with carpeting. Wood is the preferred surface. The instructor should be well-trained, and should not push you into doing more than feels comfortable. There should always be a warm-up and cool-down period for proper stretching, and no movements should ever jerk the body.

In order to reduce the number of injuries incurred by some participants, many studios are instituting low-impact aerobics, designed to be more gentle. In any case, make sure the class you choose is right for your current level of fitness. There is a vast difference between a beginning stretch class, and a ninety-minute advanced aerobic workout.

One more word about these classes or any other activity in which you engage. Two people can do the same routine and leave thinking they got the same benefits, but if one gives it every-thing he or she has, doing each movement with as much energy as possible (never pushing beyond personal limits or level of fitness, of course) and the other participant merely goes through the motions, the value received and the calories burned will be very different indeed.

I have observed that those who really intend to give the most of themselves to the class usually find a spot in the front, close to the instructor, while others move to the rear, as though they want to fade into the background, and just "get through it." Even if you aren't yet pleased with how you look in a leotard or shorts, make a decision to get the most from the time and money you are spending. Move to the front of the room and give it your all. Here comes the cliché: like everything in life, you get back what you put in.

Other Kinds of Dancing

Almost any kind of dance is an especially pleasurable form of exercise. People must respond on a very primitive level because some form of dancing is a part of every culture, from stone-age tribes through the classic minuet and on to today's rock.

There is a tremendous joy to be found in expressing oneself through body movement, to the accompaniment of music. I don't know the reasons, but I'm convinced that in most cases women would simply love to be taken out dancing, and it's the men who are reluctant to go! Maybe one explanation for the great popularity of aerobic dance classes is that you have the fun of moving your body to music, and are in effect "going dancing."

Think about incorporating some kind of dance into your life. Folk or square dancing is fine, especially if you can keep moving non-stop for at least thirty minutes. Try an evening of rock or a return to the swing era. Or close the door, put on some loud music, and DANCE! You'll feel like you did as a child, when moving your body was a joyous thing to do.

Exercise Bicycles

My current favorite form of cardiovascular activity is the computerized exercise bicycle. Some of the trade names are Lifecycle, Heartmate, and Aerobicycle. Comparing these cycles to the old stationary bicycles is like comparing a horse and buggy to a limousine.

Instead of a "straight ride," the bicycle simulates hills, so the level of resistance varies. You are given a continuous readout of information on a kind of computer screen, such as how many calories you are burning and how many miles per hour you are traveling. The best part is that you can read, listen to the radio, or even watch television while exercising, so the time goes by rather painlessly. I am so used to reading the paper while on the bike every morning, that I can't picture finding out what's going on in the world without my legs moving!

The bicycles pose virtually no risk of injury. Since you have control over the duration of the workout and the degree of difficulty, bicycles can be used both by absolute beginners and highly trained athletes. Because the bicycling is done indoors, the weather is of no concern. The major drawback is the cost. Most start at over $1,500; therefore they are not a casual purchase for the home. But these days, almost every health club has many of the cycles as an inducement to joining. It may be worth the membership fee just to have access to this convenient, efficient way of exercising.

Stair Climbers

StairMaster®, Lifestep® and other stair-climbing machines are coming on strong at many health clubs. You use your powerful thigh and leg muscles, yet since your feet never leave the pedals, you are not subject to the stress of running. Variability of settings permit use by beginners and top athletes.

People must be seeing good results and enjoying the aerobic workout, because these machines are in high demand. I have been using the StairMaster three times a week, and I think it's excellent. (To buy one for your home, you'd have to spend about $2500.)

Treadmills

Treadmills are another increasingly popular, relatively safe way to do your cardiovascular workout. You can start off at a slow walk at floor level, and progress all the way to a demanding run up an incline. (Home purchase prices start at about $800.)

Swimming and Other Water Activities

Almost everyone loves to frolic in the water, but not many people do the laps necessary to achieve a real cardiovascular workout. Swimming has a few other drawbacks. First, you must have access to a pool (or other body of water) on a consistent basis, and in all kinds of weather. Since swimming is not a weight-bearing exercise, it is not effective at warding off the onset of osteoporosis. (Then, of course, there is the problem of redoing your hair each time you swim. I don't think a really protective cap has yet been invented.)

On the plus side, swimming is an exceedingly pleasant thing to do, and is virtually free of the risk of injury (with the exception of "swimmer's ear," or too much chlorine in the eyes). If you swim continuously, you will tone the muscles, and get a good aerobic workout. Since the body is bouyant in the water, people who are out of shape or handicapped often find swimming easier than exercising on land.

There is a great deal of interest in a new kind of underwater activity—described as the ultimate low-impact sport. People are "jogging" through the water, being supported by various devices that keep them from sinking. Athletes who have sustained injuries, pregnant women who don't want to jump around too much, and people who are very overweight or have arthritis are among those who are using this method to achieve cardiovascular benefits without the risk of hurting themselves.

Muscular Strength

Weight Training

The coming trend in the fitness field appears to be weight-training. It used to be a sport relegated to beefy looking men hoisting weights in seedy, smelly gyms. Now a surprising number of women have begun to participate and in radically changed surroundings. Every sleek new health club offers free-weights (like barbells) and many different kinds of exercise machines (Nautilus, Universal,and Paramount, to name a few) for both men and women.

The most difficult part of participating in these activities is getting started. When you first see the intimidating array of machines on the gym floor, they look like devices from the Spanish Inquisition. No one should try to use them without getting proper instruction from a well-trained person. It takes a little time, so be patient with yourself. Once you learn a few simple techniques, you have at your disposal an effective system for shaping and strengthening any muscle group.

Most women sadly neglect their upper bodies. Even if they are runners or walkers, their arms are weak, and the flesh of the upper arms begins to hang much too early in life. (I was at Giorgio's one day, and heard a well-dressed woman telling her friend that she really liked a certain glamorous evening dress, but couldn't wear it because her upper arms sagged. The woman looked to be barely in her forties. That is much too young to give up a whole style of dressing, for a condition that you can do something about.

Weight-training does seem to be the fastest, most effective technique to shape and tone the upper body. Not only can you develop and firm the arms, but by concentrating on the muscles around the breasts you really can improve the bust line. While the actual breast tissue is not affected, all the supporting muscles get stronger and you can really see the difference. (Please, ladies, trust me on this one!)

The muscles in any part of the body can be shaped and strengthened with weights. Men can create a virile looking physique that makes them look stronger and feel more attractive—chests get broader, waists narrower, legs firmer. Men of any age feel young and strong again when they see muscle definition they've missed for years, or have never seen before.

You might want to look into the possibility of using ankle or wrist weights to add to the resistance of any exercise. These can be bought at sporting-goods stores. Some people use the ankle weights when they are doing leg exercises, and many walkers and runners use wrist or hand weights as they stride along.

Weight training can give both men and women a new sense of power. It is a wonderful feeling to be able to carry your own luggage if you need to, or pick up a child or a grocery bag with ease. An added benefit is that physical strength seems to spill over into the emotional realm, making you feel generally more independent and competent to handle any of life's situations.

I used to exercise with a nurse who told me that she wanted to leave a bad marriage for years but couldn't muster the courage. Weight-training and physical conditioning (and the confidence that came from being fit) eventually generalized into a feeling of power and control, enabling her to make the move toward a healthier future.

Flexibility

Stretching

Flexibility and suppleness can be maintained by regular stretching before and especially after your cardiovascular workout.

Stretch gently, flexing muscles from head to toe. Your aim is to elongate the muscles and keep the joints flexible. Stay controlled, don't force anything. Notice how every day you can stretch a tiny bit further. Remember, a flexible body is a young body.

Yoga

While no substitute for aerobic activity, yoga offers a gentle way to stretch and tone muscles while increasing flexibility. Practitioners report that deep breathing and relaxation alleviate anxiety and create calm in a hectic day.

For people who have not exercised in a long time, taking a yoga class might be an appealing, non-threatening way to start.

Spot Reducing

We'd better clear up the subject of spot reducing. *There is no such thing.* Neither doing 500 sit-ups daily, nor any amount of weight-training will get rid of the spare tire around the middle, or the saddle-bags on the thighs. What they **will** do is firm the muscles **under** the fat.

I am very much in favor of floor exercises and weights for shaping, firming, and toning muscles, and feel both are a valuable part of anyone's fitness routine. But the fat under the skin is part of the whole body system, and the only way to get at it is through sustained, cardiovascular activity, using the large muscles of the legs and buttocks—back to walking, running, cycling, swimming, rowing, etc.

Health Clubs

While fitness and a slim body can definitely be achieved without becoming a member of a health club or gym, if finances permit, think about the possibility of joining one. You will have access to the computerized bicycles, the weight-training machines, perhaps a swimming pool, and usually a sauna and whirlpool for relaxing muscles after a workout.

Most clubs offer a full schedule of aerobic dance and stretch classes, usually co-ed. They have been called the singles bars of modern times. Even if you have no interest in that aspect of club life, you will have the opportunity to be around like-minded people. Some of them may be a bit narcissistic, but like you, they are interested in improving their bodies.

Be very selective when choosing a club. Tour every one in the area where you live or work, and ask for a free trial session. Be sure to check out the facilities AT THE TIME YOU WILL BE USING THEM. A club that is almost empty at 2:00 P.M. can turn into a veritable zoo at the prime time hours of five to seven in the evening. If you want to exercise before work, make sure that the facility opens early enough. Look carefully at the other members, and see if they are the kind of people you would feel comfortable being with. Don't be pressured into signing any contracts. Take plenty of time to think over what you've seen and which club will best meet your needs.

At most clubs, there is a feeling of energy in the air. Sweating has become chic. Women with muscles are admired; men with flat abdomens are respected. This is a positive environment for someone who is rearranging his or her priority list. But *don't be intimidated!* It is not true that only lean people go to health clubs. You'll see people in all shapes and sizes. Don't wait to be fit BEFORE you go to a gym. That's like the old joke about cleaning the house before the maid comes so she won't think you're messy.

Wear sweat pants and a t-shirt or sweatshirt if you feel too fat for a leotard or shorts (many slim people wear sweatsuits too). Don't be concerned with what others might be thinking. Go in with the attitude that the only valuable opinion is the one you have about youself. Since you have made the commitment to become slim and fit, and ARE IN THE PROCESS OF TAKING ACTION, you should feel very good and very strong. What you look like today is only a prelude to what you will look like tomorrow. Besides no one really cares what you look like. They only care what THEY look like!

Most health clubs are filled with mirrors. Consider that an asset, not a liability. Overweight people are adept at looking at themselves only from the neck up, thus avoiding the whole picture. Not looking at your whole self was an appropriate self-protective mechanism to use when you felt powerless. But now that you've seized control, and are on the way to getting slim, you will be willing to take a hard look at the job that needs to be done. And as you see changes happening in that mirror, you will be rewarded for your efforts every day.

Take Your Choice

Think of physical activity as a kind of buffet, with a variety of selections from which to choose. Pick those that sound appealing, and that will be practical for your lifestyle. It's a good idea to vary your activities, referred to as "cross-training." That way you never get bored, and different muscles can be put to work. For instance, you may walk three days a week, and go to an aerobic class two days a week. You might ride the exercise bike three days, and swim three other days. Most experts feel that a day of rest is beneficial and I agree, but I don't think there's anything wrong with a good walk, even on a "day off."

Try to make exercising fun. Pursue activities just for the pleasure of them. What did you enjoy doing as a child? An accurate predictor of whether you will stick to something is how much you like doing it. Remember to be true to yourself. If you hate getting up early, signing up for a 6:00 A.M. exercise class is a plan doomed to failure. You would be better off with one of the excellent exercise tapes for your home video machine to be used when it's convenient.

A client named David was head of his own corporation. He tried going to a health club, but found that feeling like just another fat person is a setting where no one knew he was "the boss" was too difficult. Instead, he purchased an exercise bicycle and a rowing machine for his home, and work-out tapes for his VCR. David eventually plans to return to the club to do some weight-training, but for now, this solution suits him best.

How to Begin

The first steps are always the hardest part of trying anything new, especially when it's something you don't really feel comfortable doing.

For a person with a lot of weight to lose, and/or a body that is very out of shape, starting an exercise program can sometimes seem overwhelming. The concept of having to work so hard at this stuff forever sounds like a sentence to endless hard labor.

Until exercise becomes an integral part of your life (and hopefully a pleasurable one), make only a short term commitment. Tell yourself that this is just an experiment. You, as an intelligent, open-minded person want to discover for yourself what all the fuss is about—why everyone is extolling exercise as the best way to get and stay fit and to live a healthier, longer life. Over the years, I have had a number of patients who insist they started to exercise just to prove me wrong! Now they wouldn't think of giving up their fit, active lifestyle.

Design an exercise program and follow it religiously for *just one month*. At the end of that time if you don't feel better, see your body getting firmer and slimmer, begin to enjoy the activity, and like yourself for becoming a disciplined person, abandon the plan. Go back to your sedentary behavior. All you will have lost is one month of lying on the couch.

When you have made this commitment, let nothing stand in your way. Although there are more excuses not to exercise than there are calories in cheesecake, don't use them! Don't make it an option every day whether or not to exercise. Have that decision made.

At the risk of being a bit graphic, I will use the analogy that gets the attention of participants in my weight-control classes. What would happen if you awoke one morning, yawned and stretched a bit, then opted to skip going to the bathroom for the whole day because you just felt too lazy. How ridiculous! You can't do that. Elimination of waste products is just something the body does. I want you to think of exercising the muscles of your body in the same way. It's just something your body needs, and it is necessary for the healthy functioning of the organism.

Don't make vague promises to yourself. Decide on a specific, definite program that fits in with your lifestyle, and map out your strategy precisely. Plan what days will be spent at which activity, where it will take place, how much time you will spend, what you will wear, whether you will shower at home or at the facility, etc.

How often should you work out? I would like you to do SOMETHING each day (You eat every day, why not use up some calories every day?), but an absolute minimum is three times a week. You will get better results much faster if you achieve a cardiovascular effect—get to your target heart rate—four or five times a week. Besides, you stand a better chance of ingraining these new positive patterns. Habits are created in small steps, by doing the same things over and over again.

Definitely do not be a "weekend athlete"—the person who does nothing all week, then furiously tries to make up for it with one all-out tennis game on Sunday. This sort of behavior is risky to your health and is ineffective in achieving fitness and burning excess fat.

Aim for a work-out session eventually to last an hour. Most research indicates than an absolute minimum of twenty or thirty minutes at your target heart rate is required to burn fat and increase fitness. This does not mean that you have to accomplish everything on the first day! In fact it is unlikely that a formerly inactive person could or should do an hour's exercise at first. That is merely the long-term goal. In the beginning, stop when you feel you've had enough, and always stop if anything hurts. Another good way to judge whether you are doing the right amount for your level of fitness is to be aware of how you feel about fifteen minutes after your workout is over. You should feel good, not exhausted, and definitely better than you did before you started.

The first ten minutes is always the hardest. For example, some runners are full of grumbles at the beginning of a run, sure that this time they will not go the distance. Then, just as a car shifts gears from a labored-sounding low to a purring overdrive, you too will "get rolling." Many people make the mistake of giving up before their bodies can adapt to an activity mode, when everything begins to get easier.

Always allow time for a warm-up and a cool-down. The best kind of warm-up is gentle stretching (never bouncing), plus a light form of the exercise you are about to do, so you are sure to warm up the right muscles: before running, walk a little distance; before a fast walk, stroll for a while.

After the workout, slow down and stretch again. The body really needs this cool-down to prevent blood from pooling in the legs, so don't just stop exercising abruptly and go and sit down somewhere. Your muscles will be warm now, and able to stretch farther than before. Both these stretching periods are essential for the prevention of injury, and to help avoid any stiffness or soreness later on.

Because your exercise program is for the long haul be content with baby steps while you are trying to reach the next level. You will be amazed at your body's ability to progress. I've seen women who could barely do one push up increase that number by one more a day until they could work out with the Marines! And very fat people who became winded after walking half a block, slowly work up to many miles a day.

Priscilla, who weighed well over 250 pounds when she began, increased her time on the exercise bicycle by *one* minute a day until she eventually got to thirty minutes. But each increment of just one minute was as important and challenging for her as it would be for a well-trained athlete to increase his running distance by an extra mile.

The body has an astounding ability to restore itself to health and to reclaim the shape it was intended to have. However, years of being out of condition are not going to be overcome in a day or a week. In fact, if you're out of shape, and begin to follow an excellent workout schedule, it will take about six months to achieve cardiovascular fitness. Be patient! To bite off so much that you end up with muscles too sore to do the next day's activity would be self-defeating and foolish. You are not in this to win a race, but to achieve a lean body and maximum fitness, and to do it on your own personal timetable.

Listen to Your Body

Just as the body's internal cues are of utmost importance to the eating aspects of the CNC Plan, they must be heard and heeded when it comes to physical activity as well. While I believe that an "expert" should show you the rudiments of any new form of exercise, I never want you to be a slave to someone else's "program."

For example, if you decide to work out with weights, the trainer might write on a card that you should do eight repetitions of a particular movment at each session. But what if one day you are a bit "off" and only feel like doing six? Or the days when you're so strong you want to do twelve? Who should be the final arbiter of your work-out program? You, of course. With your pulse rate as the guide, and constant attention paid to how you are feeling, you are a higher authority than any expert. Just as it is necessary to abandon any one-size-fits-all diet, have the confidence to free yourself from any external dictates about your own personal exercise plan.

The Road to Success

The scale in my health club is in the main gym, allowing me to observe some tragi-comic scenes of people in the act of weighing themselves. First, the shoes come off. Then the feet are shifted back and forth, and the indicator gently tapped and retapped, all in an effort to produce a reading an eighth of a pound lower. It is usually the most overweight people who perform this daily (or hourly) ritual, apparently unaware that after one drink of water, the hard-won "loss" will disappear.

Be smarter than these ill-informed scale-worshipers. If you want permanent success at weight control, don't look to the quick-fix, transitory reward of a lower number on the scale. Of course, in time, you will see your weight go down. But it is much more meaningful to measure your achievements in terms of inches lost and new behaviors gained. Every day that you persevere with your exercise program is a successful day. Focus on tiny improvements and little steps of progress like walking five extra minutes, or doing one more push-up. Praise yourself for taking care of your body, and know that as you start to look and feel better, exercising will get progressively easier.

Learn to love to sweat! Regard it as a sign that your body is working hard for you. Feel the perspiration cleansing your pores, and washing away years of inactivity. Enjoy feeling like a beautiful healthy animal, lucky to be alive and to have all systems functioning as they should.

Don't allow yourself to be pigeon-holed as "unathletic." If you were overweight as a child, you probably shied away from gym class, and were constantly embarrassed by being chosen last for teams. You might have decided back then that exercise was for other people and not for you. (Why do schools give instruction in such things as archery and field hockey, sports rarely pursued beyond 12th grade?)

As an adult, it's not hard to find endless reasons and excuses to prove that a person with your schedule just can't find the time to exercise. But now you know that virtually nothing must be permitted to stand in your way. There is no question that long-term *weight control requires diet* and *exercise.* If you want to be permanently fit and healthy, exercise must become a basic, non-negotiable part of your life. You probably never knew that not exercising enough or in the right way was much the same as going off to war with only half the army. Now that you do know, use all the weapons you have at your disposal.

Even when you travel, your program can go on uninterrupted. Every city you visit has places to walk or run that will be new and stimulating. Aerobic classes in another location can teach you some new moves while you enjoy different music. When you are committed to fitness, you will find a way to exercise anywhere, anytime, and will be richly rewarded for your efforts.

Feeling fat feels awful. It has the insidious effect of coloring everything else in your life, starting with your self-image. Some days you may not feel like exercising. Sometimes when you're exercising, you may wish you weren't. At those moments, ask yourself which feels worse, exercising or feeling fat.

Does Every Reducing Program Stress Exercise?

Some weight-loss organizations, bowing only to the tyranny of the scale, scarcely mention the physical activity component of long-term weight management. Perhaps they are unaware that losing weight without emphasizing exercise will almost always guarantee a regain. Or maybe the consistent failure of their clients to maintain their weight, and the consequent need to "start all over again" is the way they stay in business.

There are other organizations which classify obesity as a sickness. Many people attend their meetings for years for the purpose of discussing the various aspects of their "disease" with other alleged victims, and learn how to accept themselves as fat people. While I whole-heartedly believe in self-acceptance, self-love, and mutual support, I feel there is a narrow line between self-acceptance and taking action to produce change.

Perhaps better results could be achieved by an appropriate program of increasingly vigorous exercise instead of, or at least as an adjunct to talking. The exercise not only burns calories and increases the proportion of muscle tissue, but initiates an up-ward spiral of self-esteem from actually DOING something about a problem which must be viewed as ultimately solvable.

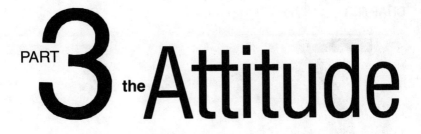

PART **3** the Attitude

7

Emotional Eating

Insight or Action?

For years, people have sought a "cure" for being over-weight through psychotherapy. There is a pervasive feeling that if only some magical root-cause could be unearthed, the fat would permanently disappear. While such explorations into self are usually valuable, they have not proven to be particularly effective in helping people to lose weight and keep it off. Even if an "aha" experience occurs—"I'm fat because I'm punishing my husband," or "These layers protect me from my sexuality"—without permanent *behavior change*, the insight is nothing more than interesting.

When I was first learning to use a computer, I kept asking "Why does this happen," and "Why do I have to do that?" Finally my instructor grew impatient and said, "Stop worrying about why—just do it!" I realized that if I had the time and ability, learning about computer circuitry might be a very inter-esting pursuit. But to operate the word processor I am using to write this book, all I needed to learn was WHAT to do and HOW to do it. I could teach myself step by step to be a whiz at operating it without ever understanding what goes on inside.

In the field of weight control too, results are achieved through *new actions*. Understanding the "whys" is less important than learning the "hows." In order to become a permanently slim person, you don't have to know why you got fat; you just have to learn not to continue doing the things that made you that way.

Some people are surprised by the concept that new actions can be implemented *before* feelings catch up. If you're waiting to wake up one morning and hear a voice telling you that at last you are ready to be fit, you may have to wait a very long time. Behavior change doesn't happen that way. Instead, each small *new action* that you take leads you closer and closer to your goal.

On a rainy Monday morning I was at the health club riding the exercise bicycle next to a group of "regulars." As we pedaled and perspired, one girl mumbled how difficult it was to get up that day. Another agreed that it was rough going this time. I felt the same way. Then the thought struck me that even though we were complaining, we were there. Instead of deciding that we didn't *feel like* exercising, and pulling the covers over our respective heads, we did it anyway. It is the action that follows the feelings that matters. We can't control what we feel, but we can control what we **DO**. As my favorite psychology professor used to say, "Only behavior is believable."

Forgiving Yourself

Hunger is a drive, but eating is a learned behavior. What you eat, when you eat it, whether you use a fork, chopsticks or your fingers are all culturally determined. The eating patterns that got you into trouble are the product of where you grew up, your socioeconomic status, and individualized family customs. You observed and learned from those around you, and sought their approval by copying their eating styles.

The first step toward change is forgiving yourself for being overweight. You are neither weak, a glutton, nor are you lacking in character. A body of evidence is mounting (notably in the work of Albert Stunkard, M.D., University of Pennsylvania, Dept. of Psychiatry) that although you have control over how your life is lived, your genetic programming may have pre-disposed you to being fat (Mayer: 1987). Even if you have no such predisposition, the chances are that you didn't always have the right information about healthy eating, and probably neither did your parents.

When you were growing up, did you know that fats are two and one-fourth times more caloric than proteins or carbohy-drates? That food shouldn't be used as a reward, or to soothe emotions? That repeated dieting makes losing weight harder every time? That exercise is every bit as important as what you eat in losing and maintaining weight? That unprocessed fruits, vegetables and grains are the healthiest foods for you to eat? Probably not. Instead of condemning yourself for acquiring too many pounds, look with pride at how much will power you were able to muster *so many different times* when you thought that dieting was the only way to get slim. Say to yourself, "I just didn't know the facts." Now you are ready to seek more effective and long lasting solutions.

When you are depressed and your first thought is of a chocolate bar, don't berate yourself for being weak. Understand that for years candy was your source of solace, and it worked, even if only temporarily. The impulse to repeat that formerly effective behavior will not disappear overnight.

Self Love

After forgiving yourself, the door is open for a new surge of self love. Become your own best friend, your own most loving mother. Be solidly on your own side, caring and compassionate. In the beginning praise yourself for every achievement, before other people notice the change in you and add their support.

Clean up your language! No more calling yourself dummy or fatso or jerk for any reason! You may be quite surprised at how many times a day you hurl this sort of derogatory epithet at the person you need to love and support the most—you.

Check your posture. Feelings about the self are mirrored in the way you carry your body and move through space. Pull those shoulders back, suck in the abdomen, raise your chin just a little. Walk proudly. Love the body you live in today, as much as you will love the leaner version which is on its way.

Do you accept compliments graciously? Most overweight people do not. The negative feelings about being fat have widened into a pervasive sense of unworthiness. When told that they are wearing a pretty dress, many women hasten to announce that it was bought on sale, or has a hole in the sleeve. When someone comments on the amount of weight that they have lost, many people will push the remark away, and quickly change the subject. It could stem from the fear that this loss, like the others, won't last, so it would be fraudulent to accept praise for an impermanent condition.

Believe in your ultimate success and your worthiness as a human being. Practice accepting compliments. Absorb them and enjoy the pleasure they bring. Your gracious "thank you" makes the donor feel validated for having such good taste, which causes even more approval and recognition to come your way.

Eating Is Not a Moral Issue

Words that should never be connected with food include guilt, sin, bad, good, weak, legal, cheat, and will power. A client named Barbara related an experience that had happened to her before starting the CNC Plan. At 2:00 P.M. after having had nothing to eat all day (mistake!), she finally succumbed to temptation and bought a croissant. She was *ashamed* of having eaten it in the car, and she felt *guilty* about having so little *will power*. After discussing the futility of fighting the hunger drive and her faulty choice of nourishment, I pointed out that anyone would have been weak with pure physical hunger under the same conditions. Making moral judgments about this behavior was and is completely off the mark.

Concepts of morality have absolutely no relevance to the subject of eating. You are an adult who takes responsibility for your actions. Foods are neither good nor bad, they are simply higher or lower in fat and calories. It is your decision when to choose one kind over the other.

Be wary of diets which say, "You may have . . . ." Who gives this permission? Who wants to be the child who must be told what to do? Who are you "cheating on" when you don't follow the rules? The decision to go "on" such a diet also carries with it the implication that when and if you go "off," you are in some way weak or failing.

This idea is the exact opposite of the Choosing Not Cheating Plan. You eat in a high-nutrition, low-calorie mode most of the time because you have made an adult decision to do so. When you choose to "be festive," you simply deviate from the plan to the extent and for the duration of your own choosing. Since you take responsibility for your decisions, the concept of guilt is irrelevant.

How to Ruin a Day at the Beach

A client named Jamie was invited to attend an old-fashioned New England clambake at the edge of the sea, to celebrate the Fourth of July weekend. Being a perpetual dieter, her first thought (after what to wear) was, "What will I eat? Should I break my diet?" Her reaction to the invitation was a vague kind of dread rather than pleasant anticipation.

The afternoon was happily spent walking on the beach, swimming, and playing volleyball. As evening approached, the aromas from the seaweed-covered food pit became more and more enticing. After chilled white wine, the great feast began: clams, lobster, corn on the cob, warmed French bread, and for dessert, blueberry pie with vanilla ice cream.

Jamie had decided in advance to be steel-like in the face of temptation. She exhorted herself to "have some will power," and to "be strong." Her plan was just to nibble the low-calorie items and resist the rest.

Need I tell you the outcome? Of course she ate everything. The food was delicious—at least everyone else seemed to think so—but unfortunately Jamie's portion was liberally seasoned with guilt and self-disgust. When the meal was over, feelings of fullness were accompanied by sharp pangs of remorse. Her self-image as a strong person had been damaged much more than her hips.

Surely something was very wrong with Jamie's approach to food. If she had been a practitioner of the program at that time, this special celebratory occasion would have been eagerly anticipated, thoroughly enjoyed, and happily remembered. She would have realized that the physically active day on the beach helped to burn up a good number of those tasty calories. The conscious decision would have been made that indeed this festive meal was worthy of the extra calories; and that she would be perfectly happy the next day to return to her more spartan, low-fat fare. Certainly there would have been no desire to continue this overeating pattern because since she had "blown it," she might as well "go the whole way."

When questions of morality, guilt, and weakness of character are removed, the task simply becomes one of balancing chosen overeating times—be they meals or days—with a baseline routine of eating foods high in nutrition and low in fat. Inevitably, equal if different pleasure will be gleaned from both eating styles.

Deciding on New Priorities

Part of taking the best care of yourself is putting **YOUR** needs first. Paradoxically, this attitude is not selfish. You must fill your own cup in order to have anything to give to others. Many of my clients are "earth mother" types, giving unselfishly to those around them, and finding *their* only pleasure in food. But in the end, martyrs and self-sacrificers are never very popular people. They and everyone around them end up feeling cheated.

Visualize a list of your personal priorities. What is of primary importance in your life? Your loved ones and your work will probably be at the top of the list. Take out some imaginary scissors and glue, and paste on top of your revised list an entry saying:

TAKING CARE OF MY BODY AND MY HEALTH

Rather than diminishing resources for the people you love and the jobs you must do, you will be creating a richer source from which to draw. An exercised, well-nourished, lean person always has more power, energy and vitality to give.

A client named Marilyn had promised both herself and me that a certain day would be the beginning of her workout schedule. But her husband wanted some information for their tax form, and her son needed help with his homework. The planned walk was set aside. It took some time for her to realize that by giving herself the gift of *time to fulfill her own needs*, she would become more effective in fulfilling the needs of others and dealing with the rest of her demanding life.

It is also important to allocate the time necessary to shop for and prepare nutritious, low-calorie foods. Don't just settle for convenience. Decide that you deserve to be nourished by the best raw materials available.

Since you put out a lot of effort, and do your best for the people around you at home and at your work—with your new priority list in mind—channel that same kind of effort and energy into taking the best possible care of yourself.

The People in Your Life

Make an objective appraisal of the people in your life. Some psychologists describe people as being either nourishing or toxic (Greenwald: 1974). If there are toxic people (unsupportive, negative "downers,") around you, consider the possibility of phasing them out of your circle. You can't change other people, but you can choose not to interact with them.

Often when you change your lifestyle, you need to find new playgrounds and new playmates. Recovering alcoholics can't associate with their old drinking companions at bars and expect to stay sober; junkies can't stay straight while associating with pushers. You may decide to trade in your old eating buddies for new friends you meet at the health club, the tennis court, or on the hiking trail. These will be people more likely to share your new ideas about healthy living.

Sabateurs

As painful as it is to realize, there are sabateurs in the world, often turning out to be those nearest and dearest to you. Watching you get thinner will make some of your friends and family uncomfortable. They see you in control of your body, and they feel guilty about not being as strong. Often they will go to great lengths to get you to eat like you once did, and to return to acting like your old self.

Someone very close to you might have a vested interest in keeping you fat. The analogy most commonly used to describe an ongoing relationship is of two people paddling a canoe. Everything goes along smoothly until one person decides to stand up. At that point, the ride becomes very rocky, perhaps even causing the boat to capsize.

If you get married as a fat person, but subsequently lose a lot of weight, all manner of changes occur in the relationship. The spouse may not want to give up the role of family "peacock," or may fear that your new attractiveness will lead you to stray. There is often a conscious or unconscious effort to restore the marital equilibrium by making you fat again. Suddenly your favorite ice cream appears in the freezer, or you get surprised with pizza or a box of candy. Now some convoluted games can begin. If you eat the candy, you can blame your spouse for your inability to control your weight. He gets his fat wife back again. The canoe is back on course.

Sometimes there's an element of competition or sibling rivalry involved. One of my clients was very close to an equally obese sister. When Laura took control of her life and began to lose weight, her sister felt threatened and uncomfortable. She launched a series of subtle and not so subtle attempts to restore the status quo—baking Laura's favorite cake and putting her on the spot about her "diet" at family gatherings. Laura was chagrined when she realized what was happening. Didn't her very own sister want what was best for her?

Co-workers will often bring especially delicious foods to the office, tempting and teasing you into returning to your old ways, accusing you of not being any fun any more. You are making waves, and nobody likes being in rough, uncharted waters.

Games You May Be Playing

Be wary of other psychological games that use eating as a manipulative tool to reward and punish other people:

• You eat to please someone (your mother, who has "slaved over a hot stove" for you).

- You don't eat to please someone (your spouse, who is acting like the policeman of your diet).

- You eat to aggravate someone (same spouse).

Don't fall into these traps. Keep your eating behavior un-contaminated by "gamesmanship." The purposes of eating are to nourish your body and to give you pleasure. Deciding what and when to eat is a private matter that should not be influenced by the opinions or feelings of those around you.

You cannot change anyone but yourself. You have just so much energy to fight the battle of losing and maintaining your weight; you must not dissipate this energy in fruitless attempts to get at the root of other people's problems and their lack of sensitivity. It would be nice if those who cared about you did everything they could do to help you in your efforts—and some will—but don't be surprised at the "hidden agendas" that may be operating when you begin to make changes in your life.

Keep your eye on the ball. Your personal goals are within your own power to achieve, regardless of the motives or actions of anyone else.

Food Pushers

It's amazing how many people will seem to take an undue interest in YOUR food. Although it is a basic rule of etiquette never to comment on what another person is eating or not eating, that rule is widely ignored by people who turn rude and inquisitive whenever they see you doing something out of the ordinary. Anyone can behave in this way, but overbearing host-esses whether family members or friends are often the worst offenders. Here are some of the typical phrases they use:

"Have just a little, I worked so hard to make it."

"One little bite won't hurt."

"Start your diet tomorrow, not at my house."

"Come on, it's a holiday."

"You're all skin and bones, you need a little meat."

It's fairly simple to deflect the assault of the run-of-the-mill pushy hostess. When offered something you would rather not have, a diversionary compliment usually works, such as "That looks great, how did you make it?" Some other responses: "I'm so full I couldn't eat another bite; I'm saving room for dessert;" or the slightly more assertive: "I don't eat like I used to." You can always fall back on the medical excuse: "I'm under doctor's orders not to eat certain foods."

With close family members, or friends worth keeping, a more direct approach may be necessary. Set up a time to talk to the pushy person privately. Use "I" statements rather than sentences starting with "you." Instead of "You always want me to eat more than I should," say "I'm making some changes in the way I eat these days, so please bear with me for a while, even if you don't understand what I'm doing."

Enlist the other person's aid by explaining that you are very determined, and would appreciate some assistance. It's always helpful to couch a request in a positive thought: "Mom, your cooking is so great it's hard for me to resist, so please don't tempt me for a while."

Confronting someone with these requests, phrased in just the right assertive, but not hurtful words, seems to be very difficult for some people. I always role-play these scenes with clients, and find it takes a lot of rehearsals for them to feel somewhat comfortable. Get another person to help you, and listen to how the words come out before you actually face the situation.

Be True to Yourself

There is a wide-ranging continuum of what each human being will and won't eat. Some people will eat anything that's put in front of them; others are strictly vegetarians; some eat only Kosher foods; Muslims eat meat but no pork; Buddhists eat no meat at all. The only important guideline for the CNC Plan is not to eat anything because of **External** pressure. Keep your own personal compass in operation and eat only what feels right to you at that particular time.

Here are some further tips for dealing with others in areas concerning food: never feel you have to justify your behavior or allow yourself to be put on the defensive. The best strategy is to deflect the question and change the subject, removing yourself from the spotlight as soon as possible. If someone says you look too thin, or that you're sure to get wrinkles from losing weight, thank the person for the concern, and ask where he or she bought such beautiful shoes.

Note how much stronger it sounds to use adult phrases such as "thanks anyway, but I won't be having any," than, "Well, I really shouldn't. . . ." By being definite in your tone of voice, the listener senses that this subject is non-negotiable. Check your body language too. Maintain a grown-up erect posture, not a child-like slouch. When offered unsolicited advice and council the very best conversation stopper is, "You may be right." Then go on with your adult behavior.

Self Talk

We talk to ourselves continually. There is a kind of tape recorder in our heads feeding us the messages that to a great extent determine our actions. Unfortunately, so much of this self-talk is negative. We are actually programming ourselves for failure on a consistent basis. Think about the type of messages you have sent yourself:

No matter what I do, I can't lose weight.

I really act like a pig sometimes.

I was just born to be fat.

I can't even control my own body.

Life isn't fair.

Whom in this world can we trust if not ourselves? So we accept all the internal messages without question, and they become integral parts of our personality and self-image. Sometimes resulting in a self-destructive, downward spiral of behavior, these negatives thoughts are guaranteed to produce negative actions. "I really pigged out today (or broke my diet), so what does it matter if I eat a quart of ice cream? I'm so fat anyway. Besides it's all the fun I have." And so overeating and the defeatest thoughts perpetuate a continuing cycle of failure.

The good news is that you can get rid of these negative tapes and their destructive messages. As with any behavior change the first step is awareness. Every time you hear one of those self-defeating thoughts playing on the tape machine in your head, push the stop button! Eject that tape! Immediately replace it with a positive thought—the image of yourself as you want to be. This substitution really works, but you must actually create some new tapes for your machine to play.

Use the Morning

The most effective time for you to conduct your reprogramming sessions is before you get out of bed in the morning. I once heard a Yoga instructor say that to give your soul time to reenter your body, you should always lie quietly for a while after waking. Whether or not we choose to believe in night-wandering souls, it does seem more gentle to awaken slowly, instead of hurling oneself out of bed to quiet a jangling alarm clock.

Lie quietly and start some very detailed visualizations. Picture yourself as a thin person in different situations: walking into the office or school in a new, flattering outfit; catching sight of yourself in profile, and seeing an abdomen that is flat instead of protruding; lying on the beach, comfortable in your bathing suit; dancing at your class reunion, the object of admiring looks.

Create new pictures every morning, and enjoy the process. These suggestions are not merely frivolous fantasy, but a valuable psychological technique helpful in the achievement of goals. Successful visualization is the first step toward successful action. You have to know where you are going or you'll never get there.

Talk to yourself in a loving, affirmative way. Praise yourself for being on the road to ending your weight problem forever and for treating your body with new respect. Think of how much progress you've made, instead of how much is left to accomplish. Imagine new cells being created every day from the nutritious raw material you are eating. Tell yourself that you are stronger and healthier than you used to be. Decide that this day will be wonderful.

The early morning is also the perfect time to tune in to how you feel. Did you get enough sleep? Are you hungry? Do you feel lean or still full from last night? What would you like for breakfast? Before the distractions of the day begin, the signals from within are stronger and clearer.

The Battle of the Inner Voices

Sometimes the inner voices in your mind seem to be engaged in a battle. One voice tells you to do what seems "right," while another screams, whispers, or whines, urging a totally different course. The tendency is to want to silence the "devil-voice"—to deny its existence and banish it forever, so you can be a permanently "good person."

This approach is not only impossible, but wrong. The negative voice is very much a part of you, and must be heard and acknowledged. If it's urging you to eat something that you don't think is right, stop and have a dialogue with it so that you can understand where the message is coming from.

Is it the deprived little child who never got enough? Is it the old you whose only source of pleasure was food? Is it just a habit that you've never stopped to examine before? End the battle of the inner voices by listening carefully to them and understanding, forgiving, and embracing all parts of your personality. In the end, you have the power to decide that the voice of positive change will be the dominant one.

Progress, Goals, and Rewards

There is always resistance to change. Inertia makes us want to stay in the same place, even if what we have been doing has not produced the desired results. But consider the simple old saying "If things aren't working, try something different." You may have tried the "lose seven pounds in seven days" approach, and witnessed how quickly the pounds came back. A more gradual weight loss is not only healthier physically, but more desirable emotionally. It allows time for you to accept your new self-image, and to actually believe in yourself as a permanently slim person.

When a dieter is asked, "How are you doing," the typical response is "I've lost ____ pounds." An answer more predictive of long-term success would be, "I'm changing my whole attitude toward eating." Learning to eat healthy foods and attaining a lean body is a *process*. Instead of scale weight, measure your progress in terms of behavior change. The first time you:

- Exercise when you really didn't want to.

- Take a bite of something, and put your fork down because it's "not worth it."

- Tune in to what you really want to eat, and it's steamed vegetables, rather than a cheeseburger.

- Leave some food on your plate because you are comfortably full.

The process of shaping new attitudes is akin to the art of Bonsai. A thing of beauty is created through patient pruning and directing of tiny shoots over a long period of time. In human behavior, an act that is rewarded tends to be repeated. Therefore, you must recognize and acknowledge the smallest achievements—the most tenuous of baby steps—with some kind of reward.

Eating is a great pleasure, but must take its rightful place as just one of the many pleasures and rewards in your life. When it has served as the sole or primary one, any suggested substitutions may sound pretty ridiculous. But do make a start at treating yourself lovingly in ways unconnected with food:

▶ Allow yourself a nap if you feel the need—many people unthinkingly eat when what they are really feeling is fatigue.

▶ Enlarge your circle of friends. Any undertaking is easier with the help of a wide support system.

▶ Buy yourself new clothes, make-up, jewelry, books, tapes, or sports equipment—anything that will bring you pleasure.

▶ Try massages, facials, bubble baths, manicures and pedicures. They offer a different kind of sensual enjoyment, and reflect an attitude of treating yourself well.

You know how difficult it is to break an undesirable habit. For some people eating too many high-fat foods is just another habit. A new behavior takes at least a month to ingrain. Along the way, think about the relative benefits of short and long-range goals and rewards.

Eating a high-calorie food gives quick "cheap" satisfaction—the fleeting good feeling you get at the moment of eating. Longer lasting, more valuable rewards are waiting for you:

▶ Trying on new clothes in a smaller size, and seeing that they fit.

▶ Hearing the positive comments of friends and relatives, and knowing they are sincere.

▶ Walking up a flight of stairs, and not getting out of breath.

▶ Hearing your doctor say you no longer need the medications prescribed for obesity-related problems (especially high-blood pressure medication).

How Change Happens

You are about to make big changes in your life concerning food, exercise, and attitudes toward other people. As with all new undertakings, you need a bit of courage to get started. Each time you have a small success, I promise that you will be encouraged to continue, and momentum will increase as you get closer to your goal.

If you have many years of damaging eating patterns to overcome, give yourself time. Ending a destructive relationship with food and substituting new, more successful behaviors is not easy. This is an evolutionary, lifetime change you are making. Be very compassionate and understanding with yourself, just as you would be to a stranger who got into trouble through poor training and lack of knowledge, but is now committed to the process of improving.

Expect to have setbacks. They are inevitable, and actually assist in the learning process by making your new decisions even stronger.

Gary stopped for a couple of donuts one evening, after eliminating them from his diet for many months. Afterwards, he said his mouth tasted greasy, and he felt uncomfortable from eating too much sugar. It will be a long time before he chooses that snack again, not because he is depriving himself, but because trial and error showed him that his tastes had changed.

Once you have acknowledged the fact that your new plan is designed for the rest of your life, small lapses are no problem. Think of them as skirmishes, having no bearing on the eventual outcome of the war.

It's true that life isn't fair. Yes, some people can eat anything and everything and never gain an ounce. It would be nice if the world were different, and everyone was given the same deal at the start of the game, but that is not reality. However, the key, bottom-line, pivotal truth is that

FATNESS IS A REVERSIBLE CONDITION.

Unlike a terrible disease for which there is no cure, your brain, mouth, and fork can solve this problem forever. The underlying message to program into your mind is that losing weight is an achievable goal. It can be done, and YOU can do it.

8

The CNC Plan

Eating Out

Eating Outside the Home

The average American eats one of every three meals away from home. Forty percent of every food dollar is spent in restaurants, and the percentage has been increasing every year. Part of this migration away from the home kitchen is due to changing social patterns—two-career families, busy lives and complicated schedules that make shopping and cooking difficult. In addition, lunch (and now breakfast) has become an important setting for conducting business.

People don't seem to mind spending a great deal of money entertaining themselves by eating. An evening in a restaurant is now *the* social activity—not something to do on the way to somewhere else. Today, there are celebrity chefs as recognizable as movie stars. Dining out in major cities has become a kind of theater—a complete evening's entertainment.

As you read this chapter, you may ask the questions: Why is this author spending so much time talking about delicious, tempting, high-calorie foods? Isn't this a diet book? What's going on here?

My first goal is to make you feel comfortable in any restaurant, whether you're watching your calories or not. But the most important reason is that you must deal with life as it really is. No matter how much you want to be slim, attempting to live every day in a spartan manner is unworkable and undesirable. The enjoyment of dining at restaurants, going to parties, attending holiday gatherings is essential to the success of your 80/20 **lifetime** eating plan.

Since the pursuit of pleasure and the enjoyment of the times that make life richer always seem to center around food (as do many business meetings) you will have to go to restaurants even while you are losing weight. You will want to celebrate events in your life. You must have a Saturday night to look forward to or the week will never end.

For years, dieters have been denying this reality. Diet books never look over the horizon to the day that the goal weight has been reached. Then what? There has to be life after diets. There even has to be life while "dieting." Restaurants and parties must be dealt with and enjoyed. When your life is balanced in the 80/20 way, they can and must be part of your life comfortably, forever, starting right now.

When you practice the plan, you will have "earned" your festive meals by choosing to follow a low-calorie, high-nutrition regimen most of the time and by incorporating exercise into your life. And so you look to the festive times with anticipation, and a feeling of mastery. You know how to live in both styles and can shift between them at will. When choosing calorically expensive foods, you always make sure that they are special and worth their cost. And of course, you won't overeat just because "this is your chance" since dining out is a normal part of your balanced life.

Fortunately, every day it becomes easier and more exciting to eat away from home, even when nutrition and being slim are important considerations. Fine dining and good health are no longer mutually exclusive. Salad bars are everywhere. Trendy, "in" restaurants pride themselves on using the freshest, most natural ingredients. Many fine and famous restaurants are successful with menu offerings under the headings "Spa Cuisine," "Cuisine Légère," "Fitness Menu" or "Lite Dining." These selections often turn out to be popular for their taste appeal, not just their low-calorie count. In such instances, foods that promote good health and those chosen simply for their taste, have become one and the same.

In some places the way food looks on the plate is now as important as its taste. Brightly colored, crisply cooked vegetables and small portions are hallmarks of "nouvelle cuisine." Heavy sauces that disguise natural flavors, and huge slabs of meat are out of current favor. You are fashionable (as well as health-conscious) when you order a salad, broiled fish, vegetables, and fresh fruit for dessert.

When you are eating out, you may opt to remain in the 80% mode—selecting foods low in fats and sugar. Other occasions may call for a 20% indulgence. The power of choice is yours. You are in control of your eating and can decide what foods you want to put into your body at that moment. The following are some guidelines to help you when you want to enjoy eating away from home, but still keep your nutrition high, and calories low.

Choosing a Restaurant

When someone says, "Where should we eat tonight?" have an answer! Don't let others take control and make the decision for you. If you have chosen to keep your calories down, most restaurants can accomodate you, but some places just make things too difficult. For example, at restaurants serving only barbecued ribs or crêpes, you would be hard-pressed to find reasonable selections.

A good starting point is to study the list of restaurants published by the American Heart Association. Serving foods low in fat and cholesterol, these places meet the AHA's dietary standards. They are more likely to cater to low-sodium requirements as well, and it follows that they are apt to be lower in calories. This list is available at no charge by calling your local Heart Association.

Do some advance research on your own as to what is available at local restaurants. Call ahead. They will usually be happy to tell you what is on their menu, and whether they will prepare food to your specifications. If you are going into a restaurant without knowing anything about it, ask to see a menu BEFORE sitting down. Many people find it just too embarrassing to get up and leave after reading the menu. They may fear they are creating the impression that the prices are too high. In

Europe, almost every restaurant—from the humblest bistro to the most elegant dining palace—posts its menu outside the door. It would be helpful if all our restaurants adopted this custom.

Getting the Most from the Menu

When you study a menu, remember the idea is for you to capture the most enjoyment possible from what the place has to offer. Neither the restaurant's menu nor the offerings of a hostess in her home are commands you must obey. Your decision about what to eat should come from inside. "What do I feel like right now, and how good is this food?" A menu is merely a set of suggestions. Don't feel you have to follow it in an orderly progression, as though it was a blueprint for dining.

If the desserts looked particularly good on your way past the pastry cart, factor that information into your internal computer. Many diners today are ordering a salad, pasta, and dessert; by-passing the main course entirely. Or you might choose to omit everything *except* the main course. Be free in your selections and unorthodox, if you so desire. Having just a bowl of soup, and saving room for a major ice cream treat may feel right at some moments.

There's a funny sounding word in vogue these days—"grazing." While the picture that flashes to mind is a herd of people, heads lowered in a meadow, the common usage refers to sampling little bits here and there. Tapas, nibbling on tidbits with a Spanish flavor at the cocktail and early dinner hour, is one popular form of grazing. I find the whole concept rather appealing, because it implies that you choose what you feel like at the moment. If you try something that isn't great, you just move on.

Being in Control

For some strange reason, we tend to lose sight of the fact that restaurants stay in business by pleasing the public. People are often intimidated by snobbish maître d's and indifferent waiters. It's time to think of ourselves as consumers. If we are not pleased, we will take our patronage elsewhere.

By preselecting which restaurant to visit, you have gone a long way toward being in control of your meal. Regardless of your choice, most places will be very accommodating about special needs. Too many people are watching what they eat these days for restaurant staff to be inflexible.

Don't hesitate to order drinks without alcohol if that's your preference. The new sparkling waters are very popular, as are some of the standard favorites without the spirits—rumless daiquiris, bloody Marys without vodka, margaritas sans tequila, a new development in non-alcoholic wines and beers with substantially fewer calories (and unfortunately in some cases less taste) than the originals. If you do order alcoholic beverages, just keep in mind that you are spending calories just as you do for food, and that the censor in your brain may fall asleep on the job.

When it comes time to order your meal, have a detailed discussion with the waiter about how the food is prepared. Your idea of a seafood salad may be cold shellfish on a bed of lettuce, while the restaurant's version may be something mashed and heavy with mayonnaise.

I was having lunch with a friend at a popular American-style restaurant. She ordered a turkey sandwich on whole wheat with lettuce and tomato. Sounds safe, doesn't it? But she had forgotten to request that it be served without dressing. Well, the plate arrived with the turkey sandwich loaded with mayonnaise, a side order of creamy cole slaw, and a mound of thick-cut, tempting-looking French fries. Deciding the whole platter looked too good to pass up, my friend ate everything—a perfectly acceptable thing to do if you are prepared to spend the calories. Just try to avoid surprises by knowing in advance what you are getting.

Don't hesitate to ask questions. Few restaurants today are pretentious enough to list their offerings in a foreign language without the translation directly underneath. If they are, make the server earn the tip by explaining each and every choice.

Most salads can be ordered with dressing on the side. Some people allow the bread to be placed on the table, but have the waiter remove the butter. (Remember, at about seventy calories per slice, bread is your friend while butter is the high-calorie food at 100 calories per tablespoon.)

Don't be shy about asking that your food be cooked in a certain way, and send it back if it isn't. If you request broiled fish with no fat, and it is served to you with a telltale glisten, politely but assertively say that it is unacceptable, and restate what you want. This occasion is no time to be "a good sport."

If you want only a small portion, split an entrée. Don't feel funny about doing this, it's a very common practice. (A few restaurants will charge a nominal fee to split the dish in the kitchen.) The "doggie bag" concept is also accepted almost everywhere. All you need to do is ask the waiter or bus boy to pack up what's left on your plate. This practice can help free you from finishing everything simply because you don't like to waste food, or because it's already paid for. You can stop eating when you are full, knowing that you will have another meal or snack for later.

Menu Clues

Here are some dangerous words that appear on menus. Their appearance usually indicates a high-calorie selection. Beware, sometimes they are couched in flowery descriptive phrases, crafted to tempt your palate:

creamed, creamy	scalloped
fried, deep fried	stuffed
breaded	batter-dipped
hollandaise	béarnaise
béchamel	Alfredo
mornay	paté
gravy	casserole
en croûte	crispy
gravy	short, rich
dumplings	pot pie
prime	flaky

ALL YOU CAN EAT

Notice how much shorter is the list of "friendly" words:

on the side	broiled
steamed	poached

Which Restaurant for Dinner?

Salad Bars

Many people make an entire meal out of a trip to the salad bar, which is certainly a healthy and positive development in restaurant dining. By emphasizing the dark leafy greens and the many raw vegetables, you are adding a great nutritional boost to your daily fare.

However, there are pitfalls. Watch out for offerings marinated in oil, especially the composed salads, like peppers and mushrooms. The garbanzo and kidney beans are a fine source of complex carbohydrates, as long as they are not in an oily dressing and are used sparingly. Sunflower and other seeds (unsalted, unroasted) can be used in moderation, but avoid adding any cheese if you want to keep the fat down.

Of course, the major downfall of many dieters who assume that salads are automatically low-calorie meals is the dressing. A couple of generous spoonfuls of a rich, oily dressing can make this meal higher calorically than many sandwiches.

Some salad bars now offer low-calorie dressings as choices, but it's hard to know what they are made of, and how low is low. Be very sparing with any dressing. Many people find that a tablespoon or less, spread over the whole plate, will give enough flavor. Or just use a squeeze of lemon or a dash of vinegar, if you don't find it too dull. Some people even carry a packet of their own special dressing, and feel perfectly comfortable about using it in a restaurant setting.

Chinese

Have you seen many fat Chinese people? Probably not. Oriental cuisines are not only among the most delicious, but also the healthiest. They are low in calories and sparing in the use of animal protein. Vegetables and rice make up a large portion of the meal, with fish, poultry and red meat used as condiments. For example, a typical serving of Cashew Chicken consists of crisp vegetables on a bed of rice, with a few strips of chicken and perhaps five or six cashews sprinkled on top.

Egg rolls, spring rolls, or anything fried should be avoided. Skip spare ribs and fatty duck. (Why the Chinese ever got the notion that rice must be stripped of most of its nutrition and made pure white is a puzzling question. But enjoy it in that form when you are in the situation, being sure to avoid any kind of rice that's fried.)

Dim Sum, little dumpling-like morsels, are widely popular among Chinese people and many other aficionados of this cuisine. I have to urge caution if you decide to try them. There is no way to tell from the outside what you will be biting into, and sometimes a language barrier precludes a full explanation from the server. Many dumplings are filled with pork and other meats, combined with exotic ingredients. Since this "foodie" wants to know what she's getting into before making the commitment of a full mouth, dim sum are not high on my list of favorites.

Soups, fish dishes, and all vegetable selections offer a wide variety from which to choose. Most restaurants offer some variation on the theme "Buddha's Delight," which is an all vegetarian dish. The sauces are usually light; in fact, when people say they don't stay full from a Chinese meal, it's because the body is not over-burdened with fat, which does, indeed, take longer to digest than protein or carbohydrates.

Although most food is stir-fried, only a small amount of vegetable oil (usually peanut) is used, and at very high temperatures. This technique prevents much absorption of the oil into the food itself. Upon request, some chefs will "stir-fry" your food in a little defatted chicken broth, avoiding the use of any oil at all.

Do request that no MSG be used in your meal. Many people are allergic to this substance, and experience unpleasant side effects. Be sparing in your use of soy sauce, since it is very high in sodium.

Desserts are never very tempting in Chinese restaurants, unless you just love canned pineapple and lichee nuts (some do offer fresh fruit). Read your fortune in the traditional cookie, and feel good about your low-calorie, healthy meal.

Japanese

Sushi (vegetables, marinated rice, and raw or cooked fish wrapped in seaweed) and sashimi (plain raw fish) are becoming increasingly popular in this country. It is very low-calorie, nutritious fare, with a couple of major drawbacks: the high sodium content of much of the food, and the question of whether some raw fish is safe to eat. On the plus side, the seaweed is full of important minerals, and the tofu (soy bean curd) that usually floats in miso soup is a good protein source, containing no cholesterol.

Almost any cooked fish or vegetable dish is fine, with the exception of tempura, which is deep fried. By avoiding that one method of preparation, you can enjoy a very low-calorie meal at a Japanese restaurant.

Italian

Almost everyone loves pasta. This staple of Italian cuisine has become the newest "in" food. It is extremely versatile, and intrinsically low in calories: one cup of cooked pasta is about 220 calories. Of course, the danger lies in the sauces poured over it. Any of the delicious creamy kinds, fettucini Alfredo, for example, are quite high in calories, while the tomato-based sauces are much lower. Marinara sauce is the safest. Chicken cacciatore is cooked with such a red sauce. Red or white clam sauces are better bets than the creamy kinds.

It's best to avoid the antipasto because of the liberal use of olive oil in the composed salad, plus the slices of salamis, cheeses and olives. Stick to a tossed green salad, so you can be in control of the dressing. Minestrone soup is always an excellent selection.

Simply grilled fish and chicken are usually available. Be wary of scampi, which is rich with olive oil and/or butter. As usual, the more composed the food, the higher its calorie and fat count will be: lasagna and veal or eggplant parmagiana are "expensive" choices.

The ingredients that make pizza high calorie are the oil, cheese, and sausage. The crust, which is just like bread, and the tomato sauce are bargains. Ask if you can have a custom-made pizza heavy on the vegetables—mushrooms, peppers, onions, and very light on the cheese, or omit it entirely. But don't forget, at about twenty-five calories a tablespoon, grated *parmesan* gives a lot of flavor without much cost.

Desserts are all pretty high in calories. Spumoni and tortoni are quite rich. If there's no fresh fruit, declare the meal over.

California Cuisine

From Berkeley in the north, down the coast through Los Angeles and all of southern California, an innovative and exciting style of cooking is emerging. Culinary trends are born, then hopscotch to New York, finally fanning out to the rest of the country.

Even the physical structure of these "California Style" restaurants differs from established norms. Leather booths in carpeted, hushed dining rooms are OUT. Now, open, exhibition kitchens are visible to diners, with tantalizing aromas wafting from special pizza ovens and mesquite wood fires. The chefs are the stars, and we watch them work.

The dining area is bright, airy, and usually plant-filled. The hard surfaced floors and non-upholstered furniture provide no muting of sound. The resulting inability to have a conversation without practically screaming is thought by many to contribute to the excitement of dining. Forget intimacy, and don't try to relate your life story, or you'll share it with the world (if they can hear it).

When it comes to food, the emphasis is on the freshest, most natural raw materials, and the use of local ingredients whenever possible. This is a boon for the health- and weight-conscious diner. Beautifully prepared fish and shellfish, crisply cooked vegetables, inventive pizzas, and exciting pastas are the mainstays of this cooking style.

Patrons have adopted a new freedom in selecting their meals. There is no hesitation about ordering two appetizers and a dessert, or a salad and a pizza. The menus and the management are extremely flexible.

Sauces are light, often made from a reduction of vegetables instead of the flour and butter of yesterday. There is heavy reliance on fresh herbs for seasoning. Goat cheese on pizza (and everywhere else) is all the rage. Salads are composed of arrugala, radicchio, mâche, and other exotic greens instead of iceberg lettuce. Sun-dried tomatoes (very low calorie, if not preserved in oil), are frequently sprinkled on pasta, pizza, and salad.

There is a definite emphasis on desserts, but not the old-fashioned variety. Today's pastry chefs compete with each other to create new, inventive temptations of all kinds: luscious fruit tarts, ultra-rich creme brulée, warm macademia nut or pecan tarts, perhaps with caramel sauce or ice cream, and always chocolate, chocolate, chocolate, in every possible incarnation.

This genre of restaurant offers the broadest latitude for your selection of foods in either the low-calorie or festive mode. I'm sure you don't need any help in the selection of the latter, so here are some samples of low-calorie, but still exciting and delicious choices:

First Courses   smoked salmon with dill and mustard sauce

mussles in black bean and garlic sauce

sliced tomatoes with Maui onions and fresh basil

limestone lettuce with snow peas, mushrooms, and bay shrimp

iced gazpacho

grilled baby vegetables

Main Dishes	mesquite-grilled fish or chicken
	pasta with tomato sauce and basil
	shrimp with papaya-curry sauce
	whole fish, steamed with vegetables
	free-range chicken, smoked over applewood
	scallops and asparagus with tarragon over linguini
Desserts	fresh raspberries
	giant-stem strawberries
	fruit sorbet
	peach-raspberry-yogurt Mousse

Cajun/Creole

This regional cuisine from Louisiana has gained popularity in cosmopolitan cities throughout the country, but seems to have passed its peak as an export. (It will never lose its appeal on its home turf.) It offers an exotic blend of complex flavors, unlike any other kind of cooking. Unfortunately, there is much reliance on deep frying, the liberal use of sausages in many dishes, and lots and lots of butter. Cajun popcorn, a favorite first course, consists of little bits of deep-fried crawfish. (The smaller the piece of any food, the more surface area is exposed to the fat, so the higher the calorie count.) Oysters and soft-shell crabs are also deep fried. The popular rémoulade dressing is based on mayonnaise. Gumbos (soup/stews) usually contain andouille sausage. The famous "blackened" fish dishes incorporate large quantities of butter with special spices to create the distinctive crust. There is a super-rich combination on some menus of tasso (smoked ham) and oysters in a cream sauce served over fettucini. (I was at a charity food tasting event where Paul Prudhomme, the famous Cajun chef, cooked this dish. It was fantastic, but so rich that a few bites were enough.)

Desserts are justly famous, but absolutely loaded with calories—pecan pie, brandied bread pudding topped with whipped cream, and of course pralines, that seductive combination of butter, sugar and pecans.

You could be quite safe ordering a cold shellfish first course, and broiled fish with sauce on the side or plain vegetable gumbo as a main dish, but you may find it frustrating to have to sidestep most of the truly representative dishes of this undeniably tasty (if not very healthy) cuisine. Perhaps if you "let the good times roll," go out after dinner and dance until dawn, you can eat everything and then burn up all those extra calories.

Delicatessen

Most selections from the deli include red meat, and are therefore high in calories. Pastrami and corned beef are particularly fatty cuts. A thick pastrami sandwich can weigh in at about 800 calories.

The one exception is white-meat turkey, which is by far the best choice at a deli-style restaurant. As long as the dressing is mustard instead of mayo or Russian, a white meat turkey sandwich with lettuce and tomato will cost only about 350 calories. Beware of potato salad, cole slaw, and any other dishes containing mayonnaise that comes along as an extra.

Chopped liver is a no-no. Liver is very high in cholesterol to start with, then it is moistened with chicken fat or mayonnaise, sending the calorie count skyward.

Last but certainly not least—cheesecake. One of the highest calorie foods ever invented by man (a woman would never have done that to her thighs). This treat can cost you anywhere up to 800 calories a slice, depending on the generosity of the portion.

Mexican

This is a difficult cuisine to enjoy if you are attempting to stay in a low-calorie mode. As soon as you are seated, you are usually faced with a basket of deep-fried nachos or tortilla chips.

At about 150 calories per ounce (just a few chips), the calorie numbers can add up before you even see a menu. In addition, many people automatically order a Margarita to complement the meal. The salt around the rim of the glass, plus the salt of the chips makes you more thirsty. Another Margarita, and you might not be quite as selective about the foods to follow.

The most popular menu items—refried beans, guacamole, sour cream and cheese toppings, fried burritos (chimichangas) and sopaipillas (deep-fried puffed biscuits) are all very high in fat.

The basics of authentic Mexican cuisine are nutritious complex carbohydrates—beans, rice, corn and vegetables. If you can order steamed tortillas (corn or flour), and unadorned beans and rice topped with lettuce and salsa, you'd be fine, but most often the beans are refried, and the rice is sautéed. Some restaurants offer broiled fish cooked in the Veracruz style, with tomato sauce. You are relatively safe with a chicken burrito or enchilada, or arroz con pollo (chicken with rice).

Mexican flan, the traditional dessert made from eggs and cream, is very rich and high in fat and cholesterol.

The only true calorie bargain on this menu turns out to be the salsa, but it's pretty hard to eat it without the chips!

French

Classical French cuisine is known for its sauces and the liberal use of butter and cream. Patés, escargots (snails) swimming in garlic butter, and foods encased in pastry crusts are just a few selections you will encounter on a French menu. Much of this cooking can accurately be described as rich, and is consequently very high in fat and calories.

The "nouvelle" revolution, and world-wide raised consciousness about nutrition and health has produced changes in French cooking. The newer versions are much lighter, with sauces made from reduced vegetables, and more reliance on natural, undisguised ingredients. But be aware that if you are dining in a traditonal French restaurant and want to keep your calorie count down, you will have to choose carefully, and ask for sauces on the side.

Cold shellfish, smoked salmon, and green salads are good starters. Stay away from onion soup becuase of that heavy cheese and bread "au gratin" topping. Avoid beef Wellington, or any facsimile, because the combination of a rich pastry crust encasing meat and liver paté is very high in calories. In fact, many of the main course selections are red meat, but you can usually find a simply prepared fish, and lightly cooked vegetables, all with the sauce you know where—on the side.

Oh, those desserts! French pastry chefs are world renowned for their cream-filled Napoleons and éclairs, iced petit-fours and custard-filled fruit tarts, not to mention rich chocolate creations. Even if you follow the European tradition of a cheese course at the end of the meal, you are still in the high-fat zone. You should be able to order some fresh fruit, or if you're a coffee drinker, a demi-tasse might add the finishing touch.

I recommend that if and when you choose a traditional French restaurant, you do so when you plan to be in the 20% mode, so you can appreciate and enjoy the artistry of this world famous cuisine, without sharply restricting yourself or the chef.

American, Continental, Chain Restaurants

This broad category encompassing most "general" type restaurants usually will offer some low-calorie, healthy choices.

You should be able to find a melon or grapefruit half, clear or vegetable-type soup, cold seafood cocktail, green salad, unsauced broiled fish or chicken, plain baked potato, vegetables, (not precooked in butter or oil), and fresh fruit or sherbet for dessert.

Be sure to question exactly how your food will be prepared. If you are unhappy with the menu, and perhaps are traveling, or with a group of people, remember to feel free to order in an unusual manner. For example, two servings of cantaloupe, a scoop of cottage cheese and an order of whole wheat toast will fortify you quite nicely. This sort of selectivity is always preferable to walking out of the restaurant wishing you hadn't eaten what you did.

Fast Food

Fast foods well deserve their reputation as the worst choices a health-conscious person can make. As one of my clients so aptly put it, fast food is fat people's food. As was discussed before, fats make food taste good, and the fast food industry capitalizes on this fact with a vengeance. Either we don't know what we are eating, or we don't care, because according to the National Restaurant Association, more than forty-five million people eat at a fast-food restaurant on a typical day.

Here is what we are eating:

> Carl's Jr. Superstar Hamburger contains eleven teaspoons of fat.
>
> McDonald's chicken McNuggets are deep fried in a fat composed mostly of beef tallow, and contains twice the fat of a regular McDonald's hamburger.
>
> Burger King's chicken sandwich contains forty-two grams of fat—*equivalent to a pint and a half of Sealtest ice cream*.
>
> Wendy's double cheeseburger, a cola, a shake and French fries has fifteen teaspoons of fat, and seventeen teaspoons of sugar.

Not only are the calorie and fat totals in most fast foods astounding, but you're sure to get a high dose of sodium and other assorted additives, like artificial colorings and preservatives.

The usual drink choices are disgraceful: coffee, soda, diet soda, or thick, rich, sugary shakes usually containing no ice cream at all. Not one contributes to the nourishment of your body or to your optimum health.

This is not the kind of food a person who wants to be healthy and slim should be eating on a regular basis. After switching to a diet that's predominantly natural and pure, these foods will start to lose their appeal, and you'll look back and wonder why you ate so many of them. But even if an all-American hamburger remains a special treat for you forever, just by cutting down on the frequency of these treats, you will be doing a lot for your health and your shape.

It is encouraging that some fast-food companies are feeling the pressure of the new nutritional awareness, and are making some positive changes. Wendy's has a salad bar, and offers baked potatoes with a choice of toppings; Denny's is using vegetable oil for cooking instead of saturated beef fat, and Burger King switched from beef tallow to vegetable oil in the preparation of its chicken, fish, and onion rings (but not the French fries). Some places offer the option of a multi-grain roll instead of the nutritionally sterile white one, and baked fish and roasted chicken instead of fried.

These improvements make eating in a fast-food establishment at least possible for an aware person. But I strongly advise you to choose other eating places until a thick juicy cheeseburger or a large order of fries has lost some of its appeal. Your goal is not to prove your will power; it is to be healthy and slim. Make things as easy for yourself as you possibly can.

"Mom Food"

A most interesting phenomenon has emerged, perhaps as a rebellion against nouvelle cuisine, with it's small portions, and precious presentation of baby vegetables, underdone fish and kiwi fruit. It is a return to the eating of the diner, or what mom was allegedly cooking in the fifties. Funny, I was around then, and I have no nostalgia for pot roast, canned vegetables, and jello molds. But I seem to be in the minority. Wherever these diner-type restaurants have opened, they seem to be wildly successful.

I hope the pendulum doesn't swing too far back. We have learned a lot about nutrition since the fifties. We know now that chicken-fried steak, meat loaf with mashed potatoes smothered in gravy, and hot roast beef sandwiches are loaded with saturated fat and cholesterol—not the foods that promote good health and long life.

If you visit one of these restaurants, listen to the fifties music, enjoy the wise-cracking waitresses, but don't let the tide of nostalgia wash away all your common sense about healthy eating.

Those Dangerous Buffets

Buffets, and any "all you can eat" situations are cues for even the most controlled, naturally slim person to overeat. There is something about all that available food that causes people to pile their plates high with assortments and combinations that have no relationship to each other. Then, of course, the opportunity to return as many times as desired is just too tempting.

At the conclusion of this sort of meal, many people feel uncomfortably full. The strange combinations are not blending well down in the stomach, and if they had to do it over again, they would do it differently.

The first line of defense is to choose another dining alternative. But sometimes, at a wedding, on a cruise ship, or in other situations, you have no choice but to visit a buffet table.

First, make an overall appraisal of what's available. Walk slowly past everything, and make an eating plan. Take small amounts of what looks particularly appealing, keeping in mind you'd like to leave this meal feeling good about your choices.

You can often find cold seafood, sliced turkey, raw vegetables, perhaps a whole poached salmon, thus avoiding the more complicated, higher fat selections in the chafing dishes, such as beef Stronganoff and chicken à la king.

If you are in a situation where hors d'oeuvres are being passed around, beware of those wrapped in pastry, or the little sandwiches with unknown filling. A few of this kind of starter can raise the calorie count very quickly, before the meal begins.

Desserts

In diet-conscious America, and especially in the Los Angeles area, desserts have never been more popular! People may be cutting down on main dishes, but restaurants have been reporting an increasing interest in ever-more inventive sweets. Perhaps diners are thinking they'd rather save their calories for something they consider a really special treat.

This strategy might help: when you're at a restaurant, and want to indulge in dessert, it's a great idea to share just one with your dining companion. You don't feel deprived, you get to enjoy the flavors, you automatically eat more slowly (so you don't appear to be taking more than your share), and you consume only half the calories.

Companies compete vigorously for the growing ice cream business. Fancy names and high prices only seem to encourage more sales. It is important to note that the higher the price, the higher the butterfat content, and hence the higher the calories. You may decide that you're perfectly happy with a non-premium brand, and save up to half the calories.

Chocolate sales increase every year. Now, instead of a run-of-the-mill candy bar, you can have your chocolate with a designer label. But no one as yet has succeeded in designing the calories out of this universal favorite. It goes down so easily, and it's so hard to stop eating. Many self-proclaimed "chocoholics" can finish a whole box at one sitting.

When the time is right for you to have chocolate, try just one or two pieces from the box, or only part of the candy bar. Take very little, savoring bites, remembering that this is not the last time you will ever have it, and that you are not a "cheater." I've heard Swiss people say (and they consume more chocolate per capita than any other nationality) that they never eat very much at one time, because it's just a regular part of their diet. (Don't forget, many Swiss also climb mountains!)

Breakfast on the Go

I hope I've convinced you that it is unhealthy for your body and inefficient for weight loss to go without eating in the morning. Finding time to have breakfast at home by getting up a bit earlier may be the solution, but if that is impossible, there are ways to eat this meal out, and still fortify yourself in a healthy and nutritious way.

The traditional bacon and eggs, white toast and coffee combination contributes little to your good health, but delivers a car-load of fat and calories. A doughnut or rich pastry is an equally poor selection. The quick "sugar high" will soon wear off, leaving you low, irritable, and less productive for the remainder of the morning.

Muffins of all types and sizes are very popular now; some bakeries offer nothing else. The problem is that many are filled with fat, sugar, nuts, raisins and other goodies. The large, tempting ones spilling out of their muffin cups can provide as many calories as a whole meal. Even the healthy-sounding "bran" muffin may have lots of shortening and sugar as well as high calories.

Calorie books are no help in this instance. A standard book lists a bran muffin as having 104 calories. You have to look closely to see that it is referring to a 1.4 ounce muffin. At these trendy bakeries, however, the big babies may weight in at eight ounces. So ask for a calorie count or at least a list of ingredients. If neither is available, use your common sense, and be careful.

Fast-food chains have entered the breakfast market, but their offerings are almost literally dripping with fat. The Roy Rogers Breakfast Crescent Sandwich with Ham, Jack in the Box Sausage Crescent, and McDonald's Biscuit with Sausage and Egg each contain nine teaspoons of fat. Picture yourself sitting down to eat nine teaspoons of fat at one meal—not exactly what a health-conscious individual should be choosing as body fuel, especially first thing in the morning.

A large bagel, smeared with cream cheese and layered with lox might be a special treat, but is too high in calories and low in fiber and other nutrients to be anyone's daily fare. Bagels vary widely in size, but a two-ounce medium one is about 170 calories. Cream cheese is fifty calories per tablespoon (one-half that of butter) and lox is fifty calories per ounce. This favorite combination for weekend breakfasts can cost you about 600 calories.

Most experts recommend minimally a cutback in the consumption of eggs because of the large amount of cholesterol contained in the yolk. Some strongly believe that they should be totally eliminated from the diet. Even if your serum cholesterol level is low (and you *should* know what it is), I object to eggs because they contain no fiber and are not a bit filling. After you have eaten two eggs and are looking around for the rest of the meal, you've already consumed up to two hundred calories (depending on the size of the eggs). You'll feel much greater satisfaction if you spend your 200 calories on a cup of cooked oatmeal and a piece of whole grain toast.

The best breakfast to have at a restaurant (as well as at

home) is whole fruit like grapefruit, orange, melon, papaya, or any other; a grain food such as cooked hot oatmeal or other cereal; or one of the acceptable cold cereals such as Shredded Wheat, Nutrigrain, or Grape Nuts. Whole-grain toast is fine, as is the aforementioned bran muffin, if you can find out what's in it, and it's not too large.

Even regular sugar-sweetened jams and jellies contain one half the calories of butter (fifty calories per tablespoon), and the new reduced-calorie kind have even less. A little spread on your morning toast can impart a real non-diet feeling. Some non-fat (skimmed) milk or yogurt will round out this breakfast nicely, but these items are admittedly hard to find when dining out.

Do keep that priority list in mind, and figure out some way—either at home or at a restaurant—to have a good nourishing breakfast so that you can start your day feeling strong.

Lunch on the Go

Lunch is the meal most often eaten away from home. You may eat in a company or school cafeteria, brown bag it in a park, have a business lunch, or meet friends just for fun.

Some people eat at their desks, but remember that a break is better for your digestion, and makes you more productive in the long run. Others conduct important business at the lunch table. This practice of "power lunching" is a part of American life, but if you will be dealing with issues that make you tense or nervous, try to arrange a non-food setting for the meeting. Food is not digested well when you are upset, and jokes about business people having to take antacids all afternoon are not really funny.

Your body functions best with a steady supply of fuel, so it's not wise to skip eating completely. Assuming you've had a high-complex carbohydrate breakfast, you will be hungry by lunchtime, but not so low and wiped-out that you will indiscriminately attack any food within reach.

Let's start with the option over which you have the most control: the brown-bag lunch. Years ago, only poor laborers brought their lunch to the work place. In the folklore of your family, are stories told of grandpa's lunch pail? Was it packed with mashed bean and onion sandwiches on home-made bread?

Eggplant and brisket on fresh rye? Meatball and pepper heros on crusty Italian bread? Cold meatloaf with ketchup on a big Kaiser roll? Most are high in fat and cholesterol, but don't they all sound wonderful?

Today, with different food choices, the noble tradition of brown-bagging has come full circle—eighty million Americans do it every day. It has even become quite chic among body-conscious people. Your portable lunch can be as simple as a container of yogurt and a banana, or it can contain a wide-mouth thermos keeping nourishing vegetable soup steaming hot to cheer you at midday.

Raw vegetables are fine, but they take a long time to chew (that's why they're great for snacks when you don't want to eat too much, like late at night), but when you're on a lunch hour, you might not get enough to eat in the alloted time. Besides, seeing anyone whip out a bag of carrot and celery sticks screams "DIETER." Since you are not one, I don't want you to bear the label.

Salads are always a possibility, but the dressing gets soggy if you don't bring it separately, and that could get complicated. You might decide to save your salads for the times you eat in restaurants or when you get home in the evening.

Leftovers are excellent for lunch. Last night's bean and brown rice combination is good either hot or cold. Unusual but excellent ideas are cold baked potatoes, yams, and butternut or acorn squashes. You might feel strange eating these in front of other people until you reach your goal weight. By then, they'll all want a copy of "the cold yam diet."

Make a whole or half sandwich on whole grain bread (or pita, which keeps everyting neat in the pocket). Add lettuce, tomato, mustard, sprouts, sliced broiled red peppers, or any other vegetables, raw or cooked. Here are some suggestions for fillings:

> water-packed tuna (with a squeeze of lemon)
>
> cold swordfish, salmon, or any fish cooked the night before
>
> sliced white meat chicken or turkey
>
> tofu
>
> lightly mashed left over pintos, kidneys, limas, or any
>   beans (just like grandpa).

Restaurant Lunches

Remember to choose the restaurant carefully if you have any control over the situation, and be specific in your instructions to the waiter.

Stay away from large composed salads. They sound healthy, but are often loaded with calories and fat. Chef's Salad has ham, cheese and hard-boiled eggs along with the low-calorie turkey. Cobb salad has all the ingredients chopped, so you don't know exactly what you're eating, but a standard ingredient is high-fat bacon. Also, this type of salad almost always has the dressing mixed in before it arrives at the table, so it's not a good choice.

Salade Niçoise has some very nutritious components: small boiled potatoes, sardines and tuna. But both fish are usually the kind packed in oil, and other ingredients include olives and hard boiled eggs. By the time you add any dressing at all, you have a high-calorie meal. There is a new offering appearing on menus lately called Chinese Chicken Salad. Typically, it contains crisp **fried** noodles, an oil-based dressing, and is not a wise choice.

If you're in the mood for a salad-type lunch, you're better off with a tossed green salad, followed by a seafood cocktail, cold seafood or sliced turkey plate (yes, the shellfish will be on the expensive side). There's always plain broiled fish or chicken, steamed vegetables, or any kind of appropriate sandwich. (For specific suggestions about what to order in different situations, please refer to the restaurant section.)

Don't ever order a "Dieter's Plate." There are few combinations less likely to help you lose weight than this bizarre combination of cottage cheese, a canned peach half, and a hamburger patty of unknown fat content.

A last word on the lunch break. If what you have been doing all morning has been sedentary, get up and move! It's good for your circulation, your muscle tone, and your mind. If you work in a big city, window shop or people-watch while walking briskly on the streets around your office.

If you can use the time for a real exercise session, so much the better. But I don't know how women can arrange to squeeze in exercise, a shower, redoing the hair and make-up, and eating a nutritious meal, all on a one-hour lunch break. Men have an advantage in this situation, and many do play racquetball or run at mid-day. But do at least stretch a little, and walk as much as you can. You'll feel revived and have a much better afternoon.

Travel Food

I am an inveterate brown bagger. Part of taking good care of yourself is not being at the mercy of whatever greasy spoon cafe happens to be located at the freeway exit.

When you're traveling in your own car, you have the opportunity to make sure that you will never get over-hungry. Since you'll surely want to take water along, you might as well buy an inexpensive portable cooler, which will keep food and drinks at the right temperature for long periods. Stock it with things like fruit, sandwiches, yogurt, and cut-up vegetables. Also take crackers, popcorn, and other munchables. (Have you ever noticed that you get hungry the minute the car pulls out of the driveway?)

If a restaurant along the way looks good, or is one you've heard or read about, stopping is always an option. Some "foodies" plan whole trips around restaurant guides. But provide yourself with the choice. Too many people have told me stories of having to eat an inferior hot dog and soggy French fries, simply because they were too hungry to wait for the next restaurant down the road.

Another good alternative is to stop at a local food store in the town you're passing through or maybe a produce stand with field-fresh fruits and vegetables. In any case, you can always come up with provisions for a picnic.

Airplane food has a well-earned reputation for being mediocre at best. With the exception of a few offerings in certain first-class compartments, and some meals on international flights, passengers are usually presented with overly ambitious but tasteless concoctions.

People are getting smart, though. Many have discovered that by simply requesting a "special meal" twenty-four hours in advance of take-off time, they can make a substantial improvement in their in-flight food. On most airlines you can choose from a selection of vegetarian, low sodium, low cholesterol, kosher, and many other meals. I have found the most reliable to be the fruit plate. They really can't do too much to ruin fresh fruit, even though for some reason it still tastes a bit "plastic."

There always remains the option of bringing your own food aboard. I do it on almost every flight. Many times, as I am enjoying my own delicious (nonplastic) fruit, a flight attendant will confide that she never eats the meals they serve on the plane if she can help it. I've heard rumors that the pilots don't either. Some people have a favorite restaurant pack a special gourmet picnic, to be picked up right before flight time.

There are airports (Los Angeles is one) that have an excellent selection of healthy foods in their cafeteria-style restaurants, but I have been in some where all you could buy was a greasy hot dog or hamburger, soda, or candy from a vending machine.

For this reason, I always carry some kind of food with me. A small plastic bag containing a high-nutrition dry cereal such as Amaranth Flakes is one idea. Dried fruits (apricots, peaches, prunes, raisins, etc.), individually packed "fruit leathers," and unroasted, unsalted nuts and seeds are perfect for traveling. They are nutritionally dense little morsels that pack easily, require no refrigeration, and can hold me for many hours if necessary. If my plane is delayed, I always know I can reach into my traveling bag for these energy-filled foods. Yes, they are high in calories, but far preferable to the salty, roasted cocktail nuts or preservative-filled cheese triangles that will be offered to you aloft.

Always carry a little something with you—in your purse, travel bag, or briefcase. You may never need it, but it's good to feel you are taking care of your body by exercising choice and control in what you eat. Even when on the road, try to avoid ever having to eat something undesirable simply to ward off the pangs of hunger.

Holidays

The very word "Holiday" has a happy sound for most of us. It implies a break from normal routine and the promise of enjoying a special time. Part of this enjoyment comes from the foods associated with the day. But sometimes, conflicts and pressures lie underneath the surface, especially if a workable lifetime eating plan has not been established. The anticipation of the festivities is then tempered by the fear of eating too much, eating in public, and the inevitability of a troublesome weight gain as a lingering holiday souvenir.

Any special times can create these feelings, but what we have come to call "the Holidays" magnifies the concerns. The season between Thanksgiving and the New Year is always associated with abundance, good cheer, and dancing sugar plums. But most people find it a difficult, stressful time. Often expectations exceed fulfillment, family gatherings produce more tension than warmth, budgets are strained, time is short, and crowds are oppressive.

Loneliness and depression are epidemic. Sometimes it seems that everyone else is having a better time than you are, with closer friends and a more loving family. Where is that snow-covered cottage in the pine trees—the one with golden light streaming from the door as grandma extends her arms to welcome you? It can be found on greeting cards but in few people's reality.

For someone trying to lose or maintain weight, the stress is multiplied. Food and eating are woven tightly, inextricably into the fabric of the holiday season. Every special day is associated with its own food or drink. Can you imagine Thanksgiving without turkey? Christmas with no eggnog? Chanukah without potato latkes? New Year's eve without champagne?

External cues urging you to eat more and in a richer manner than usual are everywhere. Billboards and televisions show glorious holiday foods. At office parties and the homes of friends and relatives, the central activity is eating and drinking. Gifts of food are popular—tempting goodies like cookies, fruitcakes and candies.

If you have a pattern of eating for reasons other than hunger, this time of year is most difficult. Emotions are often very close to the surface. Chances are that at some moment during this long season, you will succumb to feelings of depression, loneliness, tension or disappointment, and may have difficulty untangling these emotions from the old response of eating. It is more important than ever to pause before you put food in your mouth and ask yourself if you are feeding your stomach or your emotions.

Examine your traditional cooking and eating practices. Perhaps some are not sacred and deserve to be discarded. You may find that you've been eating a certain way without much thought or examination. Do you really know what's in mince pie? A standard ingredient is beef suet. Mom's melt-in-your-mouth cookies do so because they are mostly butter. Homemade gravy has about 900 calories per cup. Eggnog is traditional, but do you love it? It's "expensive" at 300 calories per cup.

Do you really want to stuff yourself so full of food at Thanksgiving, or to drink so much at New Year's that you feel sick and uncomfortable? Maybe those behaviors no longer constitute your idea of fun. Perhaps feeling in control of your body and looking lean when you greet your relatives and friends will bring you deeper pleasure.

Establish your own healthy traditions. When your children look back nostalgically on the foods they baked at your side, or those they enjoyed at the family table, let them be healthy, low-fat foods. What greater, long-lasting gift could you give them than this legacy of healthy eating.

Strategies for the Holidays

A reasonable goal is simply to "hold your own," and not try to lose any weight during this period. But you certainly don't want to overeat so that you face January 1st feeling fat and unable to get into your clothes. Here are some tips to help you:

▶ Small modifications in food preparation can make a big difference in the total fat and calorie contents of a meal:

Moisten dressing (stuffing) with vegetable broth instead of butter.

Serve plain baked or sweet potatoes instead of either kind mashed with butter and cream, or "candied."

Skim gravy as much as possible, and then pour just a tiny bit on your food for flavor.

Cranberry sauce can be made with much less sugar than called for in the recipe.

Choose pumpkin pie instead of mince pie—a major calorie saving. (Since it is a member of the squash family, pumpkin is the best bargain of all the pie fillings. Apple, cherry, chocolate cream, etc. are all very "expensive," although none is as high as mince.)

▶ The most important decision you can make is to **maintain or increase your exercise during this time.** Unfortunately, just when you need it most, bad weather may keep you from pursuing outdoor activities. But be resourceful, and keep your level of physical activity high. By doing this, you will reduce your stress level markedly, and be able to eat more of the tempting treats of the season.

▶ Don't skip meals in anticipation of a big event, allowing your blood sugar to drop and making you starved by the time you get there. But it is prudent to "bank" some calories on the day (or in the weeks before). Eat lightly, emphasizing complex carbohydrates. A good way to start a holiday morning is with an hour of exercise, followed by a breakfast of fresh fruit, a hot or cold cereal, and a little non-fat milk or non-fat yogurt if desired.

▶ Don't play will-power games. Most people have more trouble with the left-overs on Thanksgiving night than they have with the big meal itself. It you know the left-overs will be a problem for you, give them away or freeze them right after dinner.

▶ If people give you gifts of high-calorie foods, pass them on to someone else. (There are always jokes at holiday time of the fruitcake that is recycled until the original donor gets it back.) Remember, the fancy cookies that seemed harmless when delivered in the morning can turn seductive if left in the house overnight.

► Eat a little something before going to a party so you don't arrive starving: raw vegetables, popcorn, or one of the apples or oranges that are so beautiful during the winter holiday season.

► This year, focus more on people than on food.

► Go easy on the alcohol so that you don't throw caution to the winds, and end up eating more than you planned.

► Most important, keep asking yourself the question: **Is This Really Worth It?** Is this holiday food really special? If a co-worker brings that recycled fruitcake (the kind with green cherries) to the office, why bother? But if Aunt Margaret's spectacular trifle dessert symbolizes Christmas to you, then enjoy! Have the kind of fun you don't have to regret, ever.

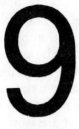

Fake It

'Til You Make It

"Fake it 'till you make it." This simple bit of folk wisdom was taught to me by my friend Sara, a member of Alanon, the support group for relatives and friends of alcoholics. The concept has sound roots in cognitive and behavioral psychology, and means that you don't have to wait for *new feelings* to take root *before you change your behavior*. For your purposes, you can act like a slim person before you become one.

The first step is to learn exactly how to play the part. What are naturally slim people really like? Do they share common characteristics? How are they different from those who fight an endless battle with too many pounds? It makes sense to identify and adopt the patterns that have made them successful. After all, if you wanted to make money, you'd ask the advice of a millionaire. With the same logic, who better to teach you how to be a permanently slim, fit person than one who is just that?

These "naturally slim" individuals for whom weight is simply not an issue are all around us, and they are the people who will serve as our models. You might even be living with one of them. Have you noticed that very often a couple will consist of one partner who is constantly battling to keep the weight down, while the other blithely eats everything and never gains a

145

pound? The slim one usually has sympathy for, but very little understanding of, what the other goes through. Somehow the pound-fighter always ends up feeling inferior—either biologically or emotionally—to this metabolically blessed individual.

Why *are* such people so lucky? Probably because of a complex interaction of factors including metabolism, self-discipline, early learning, and family styles. Broad generalizations will not apply in all cases, but naturally slim people do share some characteristics, attitudes, and actions that are worth borrowing and using. Imitating these slim people will help you to become one, and remember it's okay to "fake it" until that time arrives.

The balance of this chapter examines fifteen characteristics which many slim people seem to share to one degree or another.

1. Slim People Choose What They Eat

Slim people choose what they are going to eat carefully— sometimes spinach, other times chocolate—even opting for nothing at all if the food is not appealing or isn't just what they feel like having at the moment.

Slim people allow themselves to be "picky." They won't eat something that's stale or inferior, but will choose to wait until something better comes along. They will drive a long way to find the food that "hits the spot," whether it be the lobster served at a three-star restaurant, or the best cheeseburger in town.

They trust and don't question the wisdom of the body. If one day all they feel like eating is fruit, that's just fine.

Once they have had enough of something, they lose interest. A client told me that her boyfriend's actions once mystified her. One Saturday, they brought an apple pie back to his place, and each had a slice. When she visited him the following weekend, there was the pie on top of the refrigerator, with the same 2 pieces missing! He had simply forgotten about it. Had it been in her house, she would have heeded the siren call, and finished it to the last crumb.

2. Slim People Know When They Are Full

Slim people know when they are full, even if half of dinner is left on the plate, and the food is wonderful.

Overweight people are amazed when they see this phenomenon in action, wondering how the person knew when to stop, and what gave her the will power to ignore the delicious food still looking so tempting on the plate.

The slim person is simply responding to the internal signals of fullness that indicate when the stomach has had just enough. Sadly, the overweight person really doesn't hear these signals and will continue to eat until there's no more left.

You can observe this behavior on planes, where people will raise and lower their forks in robot-like fashion until every bite of that plastic food is gone from its plastic tray.

As we discussed in Chapter Three on internal cues, it is important to reestablish contact with the body's reliable signals. Slim people seem so in tune with these messages that they are simply taken for granted.

3. Slim People Do Not Use Food as a Substitute

Slim people do not use food as a consolation, reward, comfort, companion, or antidote for loneliness.

For the overweight person, any feeling of distress or unhappiness is perceived as a signal to eat, while slim people eat only when they are physiologically hungry, regardless of what is going on in their emotional lives at the time. In fact, when slim people are upset, they often "can't eat," and when they're very busy, excited or agitated, they tend to forget about food.

If you offered a very unhappy slim person a pizza as a consolation, he would probably think you were crazy. The response would probably be something like "Are you kidding? I couldn't eat a thing."

But eating from stress is a very common pattern. It might be the way you have soothed yourself for many years, and it probably has worked—at least for a little while. So getting yourself to make a change will take real strength.

Start by becoming aware of how naturally slim people (and animals) seem to "shut down" the desire to eat when they're tense. They need comfort and companionship as much as you do, but they look for it in places other than food—from nurturing people or activities they enjoy.

Start to model your behavior after theirs, but know that this will be one of the most difficult changes you will ask yourself to make. Until you are completely successful, switch the foods you eat at these painful times from the high-fat variety to those high in complex-carbohydrates. (Please see Chapter Seven.)

4. Slim People Take Care of Themselves
Slim people know the importance of proper nourishment, and spend time, money and energy taking care of their bodies.

It is generally fit people who are most interested in "health foods." They are very concerned about what they are putting into their bodies, and as a rule, eat fewer "junk foods" than overweight people. Study shopping carts as you walk the supermarket aisles. Often you will find that slim people are making "leaner," healthier choices, while overweight people have loaded their carts with chips, cookies, prepared foods, and of course, diet soda!

Slim people will tend to think ahead, and take care of themselves by bringing a brown bag if they are doubtful about what foods will be available at a particular destination.

A client named Gina who is a cabaret singer, reported that she had "blown it" the previous day by eating high-calorie (and bad tasting) fast food, because she was starving and it was all she could find. I asked why she didn't pack a sandwich, or at least a little snack since she knew in advance she would be in a part of town where there was nothing good to eat. "Oh," she said, "I never think about things like that—there's always someplace I can stop between auditions and grab something."

Start to take better care of yourself by doing some advance planning as many slim people do. If you don't want to bring your own food along, at least investigate ahead of time where you can buy something acceptable. It's fun to always be open for unexpected opportunities, but having a general plan about how you will nourish your body is an important, self-loving thing to do.

5. Slim People Do Not Usually Skip Meals
Slim people eat regularly, they rarely omit breakfast, and do not skip a meal to prepare for a later overindulgence.

You won't hear a slim person saying, "I'm not going to eat a thing all day, because tonight is going to be a pig-out." Since you know that saving up calories in that way invariably leads to overeating, don't do it!

Naturally slim people might eat lightly on the day of a big occasion in order to make sure they are hungry enough to enjoy it, but would never consider going without breakfast and lunch to "starve themselves" in advance.

Keep your blood sugar at a consistent level, and you will feel better, have more energy, and be less prone to overeating under any circumstances.

6. Slim People Do Not Eat by the Clock

Two people share an elaborate lunch that lasts long into the afternoon. The overweight person will sit down for dinner at the usual time, without giving a thought to whether or not he is hungry. The slim person, still feeling full, will have a big glass of water, something very light, or nothing at all for the evening meal.

It doesn't matter what time it is. How do you feel? Are you in need of fuel? Is it only habit that is leading you to eat more than you need? Let the signals come from inside you, not from the clock on the wall.

Sometimes social pressures make life complicated. Margie, a television dancer, told me that she is hungriest in the morning and at noon, and prefers to eat lightly in the evening. Her new husband has the opposite pattern. After work, they go for a run together, come home and prepare dinner. At that point, Margie feels like eating some fruit, or something comparably light. But her husband sulks when she doesn't share in the preparation and consumption of his full-course meal. When I asked her how she handled the situation, she said that her solution was to eat small amounts of the heavier food.

Because I so strongly believe in heeding the body's signals, and never eating anything to please or punish another person, we talked about other ways to handle this issue without ruining the marriage!

She was very willing to help prepare his food—she just didn't want to feel pressured to eat it. She explained this to him nicely, and continued to join him at the table as she always did. In a few days, he ceased to pay attention to their different selections. After all, when people go to a restaurant, they rarely order the same thing.

Within the limitations of schedules, clocks, and social pressures, try your best to eat what and when your body tells you to, as slim people seem to do.

7. Slim People Eat When Hungry

Slim people eat nutritious food or high-calorie food, but only when they are physiologically hungry.

Two people are walking past a bakery. The overweight person will spy a luscious looking pastry, buy it and eat it without giving a thought to the large lunch consumed an hour before. The naturally slim person will also admire the bakery's goodies, and then do one of three things: take a little bit of the friend's pastry, buy some to enjoy later, or make a note of the shop's location for a future visit.

Most slim people really do eat only when motivated by internal cues of true hunger, and never just because food is available. Because to them food will *always* be available. They never have the painful thought that someday soon they must reenter the dreaded world of "dieting."

8. Slim People Never Go on a Diet

Since overweight people know only two modes of eating, eating too much or dieting, they are alternately out of control, grabbing for all the formerly "forbiddens" (and eating them *fast*), or rigidly restricting themselves to a punitive, very low-calorie diet which must at some point end. And then what? Back to the overeating mode. The painful cycle never ends. It's a dispiriting thing to do to yourself emotionally and an unhealthy way to treat your body.

Slim people on the other hand, know very little about calories. Sometimes they eat a lot, sometimes hardly anything. Both healthy foods and "fun" foods are part of their lives. They seem effortlessly to travel a middle road, enjoying their comfortable relationship with food. That must be your goal too. Give up trying to lose a certain number of pounds on yet another diet. Be satisfied only when you too can achieve a comfortable lifetime relationship with food.

Ernie, a television producer, was one of my most successful students. Now his brother, John, is attending my class. The other evening I asked John how Ernie was doing. With a big smile, his answer was "163." This response gave me enough material to fill the whole class time.

Does it matter what Ernie's scale weight is today? Not very much. What he weighs five years from today is what matters. Instead of a response in the form of a number, I would have been encouraged had the answer been something like: "Ernie exercises every day now—nothing gets in his way. His diet is so healthy, and he doesn't get tempted by the stuff he used to eat. But when we go out, he always has a good time, and eats whatever he wants. He told me he's not afraid of getting fat anymore."

Now you're talking! These are the new behaviors that will get stronger each day. These are the actions that predict long-range success, the only kind to value. I really didn't mean to jump on Ernie's brother for his naive numerical answer, but I hope I convinced my group—and you—that reduction in scale weight is the easy part. Maintenance is what counts, and "going on a diet" for a prescribed length of time, without learning new ways of dealing with food, is an ineffective plan that will not succeed.

9. Slim People Eat More When In Public

Overweight people are often ashamed of their condition, and do not want to call attention to themselves. Therefore the typical eating pattern is to eat like a sparrow in public, but a vulture when alone.

It is at these solitary eating times that most of the damage is done. They can occur when a person is alone in the house, in the car, in the kitchen when everyone is asleep, or in a bedroom with the door closed. There is often an element of "sneakiness" in this behavior, and it is always characterized by eating fast—what some call "scarfing."

Slim people act in an entirely different way. At home, they usually eat rather sparingly, often emphasizing high-nutrition, low-calorie foods, sometimes grabbing anything that's around. But because food is associated with pleasure and fun, get them to a party or a restaurant where the food is special, and watch out!

This is a very important reversal of behavior for you to make. For the times when you are alone, decide to buy and eat foods that are low in fat, but high in nourishment for your body.

Eat them slowly. People only eat too fast when they are afraid that something or someone will take the food away. "Something" or "someone" is usually their own conscience.

Please don't label any eating as "cheating." You are an adult making rational decisions. You are aware of the consequences of eating high-fat foods, and the need to balance those times with a more spartan eating style and with plenty of exercise. When the food is so good that you're willing to pay the price, don't rush through it. You may as well savor every calorically expensive mouthful.

I became very good friends with a client named Jacqueline, who had followed the pattern of eating a lot at home, and very little when she was with other people. She had lost about thirty pounds, and was about to move to New York after spending a year in Los Angeles.

We went out together for a special farewell dinner. Over champagne, we studied the menu carefully and ordered a multi-course meal that included pasta in a rich, creamy sauce, and concluded with chocolate raspberry truffle cake. The food was extraordinary, and while we savored the flavor and texture of each bite, neither of us felt it necessary to finish everything on the plate.

We thoroughly enjoyed the food, the celebration of a new friendship, and the marking of a turning point in her life. As she openly and slowly enjoyed this once "forbidden" meal, she said that she felt like a "normal person" for the first time in a long while, freed at last from the diet mentality.

When **YOU** go out in public, allow yourself to participate in life's festive situations. You will make the decisions about whether you want to stay in the 80% mode at the moment, and/ or whether the food is really special enough for an indulgence. Make solitary overeating a thing of the past, and make enjoyment of eating in public a new pleasure.

10. Slim People Enjoy Food More Than Overweight People

A common occurrence in my practice is for a fat person to ascribe his condition to the fact that he or she "really loves to eat." I always smile at this admission, because the implication is that slim people do not. Ironically, slim people actually may be getting **MORE** enjoyment from food than their chubbier friends.

For someone with a weight problem, food has been a source of immediate pleasure, but long-term pain. Often these ambivalent feelings produce rapid, mindless eating, followed by feelings of guilt and remorse. Even thoughts of food become cues for discomfort, because they have led to overeating, and eventually to being fat. So while slim people welcome them as a prelude to pleasure, overweight people want to push food thoughts away.

While there are a few skinnies in the world who seem genuinely uninterested and eat only to live, most normal-weight people spend a great deal of time not only eating food, but thinking about it, and planning what and where to eat next. They subscribe to gourmet magazines, love to try new recipes and restaurants, and can describe a favorite meal in exquisite detail. Vacations and trips may even be planned with special foods in mind.

Strikingly slim Helen Gurley Brown, editor-in-chief of Cosmopolitan Magazine, wrote that while her producer-husband was busy at the Cannes Film Festival she was preoccupied with decisions of which restaurants to visit in the bountiful countryside of the south of France. (But she also writes of being totally dedicated to her exercise program, and of carefully watching her diet most of the time.)

Since slim people usually eat more slowly, there is extra time for the perception of taste and thus greater enjoyment of flavors and textures. An overweight person will have finished off an ice cream cone long before his slim friend has licked around the sides. These dawdlers are having a wonderful time, while the fat person is left frustrated and wanting more.

It's okay to love to eat! It's natural and right, and the way things are supposed to be. A healthy person is blessed with a good appetite which, when channeled properly, can bring pleasure as well as nourishment at least three times a day.

11. Slim People Make Exercise a Priority

Slim people work their schedules around exercise, because it has a high priority in their lives.

154 *The attitude*

Have you heard the expression "last hired, first fired?" It means when it's time for layoffs it's the new people—those with the least seniority—who go first. There are similarities in human behavior. When a habit is brand new, it's like a fragile pale-green blade of grass, easily trampled or uprooted. Later, when it has grown strong and established, it can withstand a heavy storm.

When you have just begun to exercise, and it doesn't yet feel like a natural thing to do, the slightest excuse will be enough to make you change your plans. My client Marilyn said she couldn't go for a walk because it was raining. But it was a gentle, misty rain, and wouldn't have stopped a person for whom exercise was a routine part of life.

Suzanne had just begun to exercise regularly when she and her husband went to a northern state to visit his parents. It was too cold to run, she reported, and she didn't know what else to do, so she gave up physical activity for the week.

I asked her to play a game with me. What if someone had told you that you must exercise this week or die. What would you have done? She thought for a moment, and then said that she would have gotten out the yellow pages of the phone book, looked up exercise studios and gyms, found a local "Y" with a swimming pool, walked briskly in the snow, volunteered to shovel the front walk, or worked out to music from the radio. In other words, she would have found a way.

Many slim people have become very resourceful in making sure that their exercise can continue in an uninterrupted manner whatever the weather, wherever they travel, and no matter what is going on in their lives. While others try to "work it in," those who are committed make it a priority. When visiting a new city, they will carry with them the names of the best restaurants in one hand, and a list of hotels with health spas, or parks for walking or running in the other.

12. Slim People Use Exercise as a Tension Reliever

When an overweight person is tense or worried, eating is usually the activity of choice, but in the same situations, a naturally slim person will often turn to exercise. When a slim person is agitated, he or she will become fidgety, and be unable to sit still. Pacing the floor is more common than curling up in a corner or sitting immobile in a chair. You hear about these people taking a brisk walk to "clear their head."

Since movement is the healthiest, most effective way to react to stress and provides the greatest relief, it is an excellent behavior to borrow. But it's going to feel decidedly wrong at the beginning. You want to fill the aching hole inside you with rich delicious food, and instead you're supposed to go for a walk, a swim, or a bike ride. How ridiculous! But if you do it once—just once—you start an upward spiral with great implications for your future.

First of all, a lot of tension will actually be drained away by vigorous body movement. Even more important, you will return home with a net calorie loss instead of a huge eating episode to feel guilty and remorseful about for days. You'll be filled with good feelings about yourself. Since any act that is rewarded tends to be repeated, you stand a good chance that the next time you are under stress, you will exercise instead of eat. What a dramatic change for you!

There was a particularly stressful time in my life a few years ago. I was doing my usual morning exercise routine, but by late afternoon, the calming effects had worn off. I would feel myself getting restless, and I knew that it was time to drop everything, get out of the house and MOVE.

At that time I lived in La Jolla, California, near San Diego, one of the most scenic spots on the Pacific coast. Many times I drove down to the little village, parked my car, and walked as fast as I could up and down the hills around La Jolla Cove. The setting was beautiful, but I wasn't seeing it at those times. I would stride along for about forty-five minutes, sometimes thinking about problems, other times trying not to think at all.

By the time I walked back to the car and drove home, my body was tired, but I didn't feel tense any more. Physical fatigue seems to be incompatible with mental stress. No facts of my life situation had been changed; no circumstances improved. Only my state of mind had been altered.

I still find that the most effective thing I can do when I feel unhappy is to get up and move. It really helps me, and I want it to help you too.

13. Slim People Know When They Are Eating

Slim people don't eat unconsciously, without awareness of what they are doing. After being on the telephone or while watching television, they never find themselves with a mysteriously empty cookie box or can of peanuts by their side.

In many behavior-modification programs, the first assignment is to write down each bite of food that goes into your mouth. You must count every little taste, chance nibble, the leftovers you finish from your child's plate, and even the times when you stand in front of the freezer and have a sliver of cheesecake just to even it out!

If you suspect that you are doing some unconscious "grazing," try logging exactly what and how much you eat, what time of day it is, and what your emotional state is at the time. You may be surprised at what you'll discover.

For instance, you may realize that tasting dinner all through the cooking process is in effect eating two whole meals; or that going through the bowl of mixed nuts at cocktail time computes to a huge calorie outlay.

Being aware of everything you eat is the key to control and making wise choices. You wouldn't just throw money around without knowing what you were buying. *Every* calorie should be wisely spent. Certainly if you're going to eat high-calorie foods, you might as well be fully conscious of the experience!

14. Slim People Do Not "Believe In" Will Power
Slim people think that will power—resisting food when you are truly hungry, is a ridiculous concept.

People who are fortunate enough to be unconcerned about calories are often amazed at the self-denial practiced by their "dieting" friends. The process seems so simple to the lean ones—when you're hungry, you eat.

It is interesting to note that some slim people actually find a kind of enjoyment in the state of hunger at certain moments. They report feeling lean and powerful, and very much in control, perhaps because they know they can choose to eat at any time.

That, however, is a very advanced concept! For people with a long history of weight problems, the wisest thing is to switch to a high complex-carbohydrate diet, so that low-calorie, high-fiber, filling foods keep the pangs of hunger away. This is a healthier, more humane road to take than trying to eat half as much of the high-fat foods you used to eat. Also remember to rid your surroundings of high-fat foods. Don't tempt yourself, and then try to exercise will power. Make your life easier, not harder.

15. Slim People Are Very Disciplined

It is not uncommon to see people take the same parking space, the same locker, and the same exercise bicycle every day; play racquet ball with the same partner on the same court three times a week; or walk each morning at a particular time, rain or shine. (My father weighs himself each year on his birthday, and makes sure that the number is the same as it was the previous year.)

Yes, these people are showing rigidity, consistency, or discipline. Call it what you will. But it does seem to be a critical element in the ability to control weight. It's a good idea to use people like this as role models in this regard, since discipline is a trait sometimes deficient in the overweight.

Even if you are a free spirit in other ways, model the behaviors of slim people in the areas of exercising and eating. Stick to your exercise schedule, even at times when it's a push. Develop the discipline not to eat the food in front of you if it's not very good, or isn't really what you want.

Be tough on yourself, but be the same on your role models. Demand excellence. I wouldn't attend the aerobics class of an instructor with less than a great body; nor would I go to a doctor who was fat, out of shape and smoked cigarettes.

When you are choosing a physical activity, take a long look at the practitioners of that sport. If you admire the swimmers' body (broad shoulders, narrow and lean at the hips), and are turned off by the concave look of some long distance runners, take these factors into consideration. If someone is giving you dietary advice, look very hard at that person, and see if the advice has worked for them.

Once you open your eyes to the activities, attitudes, and techniques used by people who are successful at what you want to do, blatantly, freely, unabashedly copy them! Learn everything you can about what they do and how they feel. Ask questions and follow their advice.

These steps will be a shortcut to your own personal success, and one day, to your surprise, you'll find that it all feels very natural, and that you don't have to fake it anymore.

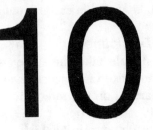10

Choosing You:

A New Image

Am I Fat, and Are You Fat?

Now comes a legitimate question, "have you ever been fat, Midge?"

Just enough. While I believe that you don't have to experience something in order to understand it—male obstetricians deliver babies, and psychologists treat disorders they've never had—my short period of having extra poundage as a teenager made me understand what it was like to be unhappy with my body. Really obese people may find it hard to believe, but when a naturally slim person gains a few pounds, their clothes don't fit and there really is "nothing to wear." At this point their self-confidence plummets, the feelings of self-disgust are very real, and cause the same kind of pain as does the fifty pounds someone else needs to lose. The feelings are universal. Only the numbers vary.

I live the 80/20 way every day, and so do my clients. In an area where successes are very limited, most of my clients have mastered their weight problems. I hope you view this track record as my credential for being able to help you become fit and stay that way for life.

You may have noticed that all through this book, I don't use very many expressions about people being FAT. I thought a lot about this, and decided the reason is not a euphemistic desire to cover up the situation with more pleasant words. It's just that I don't really picture anyone **AS** fat—or believe that anyone **IS** fat. In my mind, the person **HAS** fat—a burden that the person is **temporarily** carrying around, a burden that eventually can be laid down.

A wonderful expression used in reference to handicapped people is that they are temporarily inconvenienced. That's how I feel about the condition of fatness. But unlike some other handicaps, this one is reversible. Fatness can be permanently overcome.

I want you to separate yourself from the extra load you are carrying. The real you lives somewhere deep inside in a perfect inner core that is forever lean and beautiful. Your job, at once simple and complex, is to pare away the layers so that this person can emerge. You are not fat. You *have* fat. Now you have learned how to get rid of this temporary inconvenience. Make the important decision to lay your burden down.

Choose To Be Slim and Healthy For Life

When asked how he feels, my terrific father (who has passed his 80th birthday) usually replies that he is "splendid." But that response is hardly universal. Some people have strayed very far from the ideal condition they were meant to enjoy. They think that constant unsuccessful dieting, sluggishness, lack of energy, dependence on antacids, laxatives, stimulants and relaxants are just part of life. But barring accident or illness, feeling SPLENDID should be the norm. Not all the time, not every moment of every day but the baseline health condition of a human being is supposed to be **HIGH-LEVEL WELLNESS.** This phrase implies so much more than the absence of sickness. It encompasses a feeling of well-being, of energy, of youthful vitality and of being comfortable inside your body, proud of the way you look.

The human body is brilliantly designed. Being lean is the way you're *supposed* to be. Remember that we are all animals and the only other fat animals are in zoos or living in homes as people's pets.

In our modern society, people have a tendency to be overly intellectual and to neglect their bodies. After all, with the exception of professional athletes, most of us get ahead in the world by using our brains. But our "self" is very much a "body" too. Often the body is taken for granted, not treated with the appropriate respect and love. Sometimes we act as if our "body" is indestructible (especially when we are young). We abuse it with smoking, caffeine, drugs, alcohol, stress, lack of sleep, insufficient exercise, too many unhealthful foods, and with excess weight.

We are made aware of this neglect from little things: the sudden realization that there is a good amount of flesh to be pinched at our waistline, or that our breathing becomes labored after walking up a flight of stairs.

Sometimes our need to accept our physical natures is brought home when suddenly we suffer a heart attack or stroke. Or, we find ourselves sitting across the desk from a somber doctor who has diagnosed a potentially life-threatening condition.

In an ideal world, the human animal wouldn't need such traumas to change old ways. Many times, however, a catalyst does seem to be necessary. Sometimes there is no jolt, just quiet desperation, because nothing has worked no matter what we have tried in our efforts to lose weight. Regardless of how you reached **your** turning point, decided to improve your health and become fit **permanently,** the important fact to remember is that the human body has an amazing ability to withstand the abuse of many years and, barring illness, the potential to reverse damage already done. Your body has just been waiting to be cared for properly, and it will reward you with better health and a lean new shape.

Food has been and must continue to be a great source of pleasure in your life. The underlying concept of the Choosing Not Cheating Plan is that being slim and well-nourished *and* eating for fun are not mutually exclusive. But think for a moment: the real purpose of eating is to build and maintain cells, to give your body the energy to live, to nourish you and sustain your life.

After traveling through the incredibly complex digestive system where each organ and enzyme plays a crucial role, the food you eat actually becomes a part of you. Each one of your cells, knowing what it needs to build skin and hair, repair muscles and kidneys, fight infection and disease, picks up exactly the right combination from the blood stream. It's really a kind of miracle that what you eat turns into YOU.

Having new respect for your body will lead you to more thoughtful food choices. It stands to reason that the best raw materials create the strong healthy body you would like to inhabit—the one best equipped to ward off sickness, be filled with energy and stamina, and most able to live fully at any age. These choices help you, also, to look your very best. There is a different standard for beauty these days. The emphasis is no longer on being skinny, but on being healthy looking and fit. Yes, beauty means being slim, but it also means glowing with vitality.

Increasingly research shows that being and staying healthy is not our doctor's but our responsibility. The fountain of youth and health may very well be inside us. We have no power at all over many of life's misfortunes, but we do have ultimate control over what we eat, and hence, quite literally, of what we are made.

Guess what the bonus will be when you follow the right diet for good health and long life? That's right, it's being slim. Permanently. The same diet for good health is the most effective diet for losing fat and getting down to your ideal weight and staying there. Reaching a state of high-level wellness brings an added dividend: the slim body you've been seeking for so long.

Start Today

Even if you don't "feel" ready, start anyway. Let the positive cycle begin. Even the smallest step is the beginning of a unity of lifestyle—a circle of health: If you start a walking program, you're outdoors in the fresh air and sunshine. You feel less stress, appreciate nature more, become more in tune with your body. After virorous exercise you just don't feel like lighting a cigarette or eating fatty foods, so your weight loss accelerates. Since you are lighter, you can walk with greater ease and pleasure, so you tend to do it longer and that makes you lose more weight. You buy new clothes and feel proud, so your posture gets better. People start to notice. You're rewarded for taking care of yourself, so you continue to do it. You're on your way.

Have No Regrets

A long time ago I read a quote that has stayed in my memory. A very thin old woman was asked if she had any regrets in her life. She mused a moment and then replied "Yes. I should have had more ice cream and less beans."

Of course that story can be interpreted on two levels—first, as a metaphor for life: We have so little time, we'd better get the maximum enjoyment from living that we can, so we don't reach the end of the road filled with the pain of regret.

On the more literal level, of the foods you choose to eat over a lifetime, it seems equally sad to look back on high points, special moments, times of celebration, and remember feeling deprived, frightened about eating too much and gaining weight, never allowing yourself to have the fun of eating that others seemed to have so naturally.

But let's look at the other side. Picture an overweight, under-exercised patient who has just suffered a heart attack. While lying in his hospital room, tubes attached to every orifice, he is probably regretting the many ways he abused his body— the years of eating high-fat foods, carrying around too much weight, making his heart work too hard—years of smoking and drinking to excess. He is no doubt making fervent promises to live in a more healthful way if only he's given one more chance.

Or, think of a woman who has been fat most of her life, fighting the endless battle, always feeling like a failure. Getting old without ever being able to fit into the clothes she has always wanted to wear, or having the pleasure of seeing herself as a slim person.

Somewhere between these examples lies the road to a life of moderation—of selective enjoyment—informed indulgence, pure pleasure from eating and drinking, combined with exercise, and a home-base style of high-nutrition, low-calorie eating.

The way to reach this ideal middle ground is by making *fundamental*, irrevocable changes in your lifestyle. Certainly, no temporary "diet" is of any value. Indeed, no one diet can be right for everyone. But everyone must establish a healthy, comfortable relationship with eating. Because unlike dealing with alcohol or drugs, no one, no matter how overweight, can abstain from food and go on living. And no one, no matter how motivated, can swear-off eating for pleasure and ever succeed in the long run.

You have to pay your dues. Eternal vigilance is not only the price of liberty, but of a fit body. You must view your exercise program as a necessary, "organic," continuing part of your life. You must eat in a high-nutrition, low-fat style most of the time, and choose your times of indulgence wisely.

The successful formula is quite simply the 80/20 Choosing Not Cheating Plan. I hope you choose to live by it so that you do not suffer either the regrets of overweight people or of the deprived woman described above, but feel you have successfully balanced all the needs in your life.

Now it's time to take the leap, and begin the process. There are few guarantees in life, but if you follow this program, I can absolutely guarantee that you will lose weight and feel better. I know you can do it. And you know you can do it. All you have to do is begin. Why not right now?

PART 4 the Appendix

11

What You Need
To Know

About Nutrition

Nutrition is an infant science. Few people know much about it, but everyone is happy to offer an opinion. New, often contradictory research is reported every day. How can a non-scientist make intelligent decisions about what foods to eat when the experts so often disagree? More disheartening, new information contradicts the old, pointing out that we have been doing everything wrong up 'til now!

How then can the average person, concerned with good health and wishing to be slim, intelligently select a framework on which to build a lifetime eating plan? One that will withstand attack from the new and unproven, the latest fad and extravagant promise?

The decision might be easier after a quick study of the structure of our bodies and our history as a species. These are the bedrock foundations upon which I have constructed my personal approach to food, and the one I recommend.

The facts are that the human body has not significantly evolved since its primitive origins millions of years ago, but what we in modern civilization put into that body is drastically different. As a consequence of these dietary changes, we are prone to obesity and a host of other degenerative diseases, now irrefutably linked to the foods we eat. Cancer, heart disease, diabetes, and high blood pressure have displaced infectious diseases as the great scourges of humankind.

To help uncover some of the causes of this predicament, it is instructive to think about what primitive people were *not* eating.

What Our Ancestors Did NOT Eat

An Overabundance of Animal Protein

Primitive man was an opportunistic meat eater. Only on the occasions when a kill could be made or a fish caught was flesh consumed. No one was having bacon and eggs for breakfast, a hamburger for lunch, and a steak for dinner. In addition, the animals that were eaten were not fattened on feed lots, locked in restrictive cages, or innoculated with hormones and antibiotics. Todays bred-for-food animals are very different from their free-ranging, lean ancestors.

Processed Foods

A fruit was eaten in its whole form, not squeezed to extract juice, leaving the fiber and many nutrients behind in the pulp. A grain wasn't stripped of its outer bran coating and vitamin-rich germ to make a "refined" product. An olive was not transformed into a bottle of oil. A potato was a potato, not a French fry, chip, or flake.

Excess Fats

Meats were not "marbled" (richly endowed with fat). There was no butter, margarine, oil, or cheese readily available in convenient packages. Of course, there were no fried foods. This tasty but hypercaloric method of food preparation had yet to be invented. Here is the "progress" we have made since then:

8 oz. baked potato	160 calories
8 oz French fries	620 calories
8 oz. potato chips	1200 calories

Refined Sugar

Refined sugar was unknown until the eighteenth century. Now, sugar-laden cakes, pies, and candy assault the same model pancreas that was structured to metabolize something only as sweet as ripe fruit or occasionally honey. The average American now eats over 120 pounds of sugar per year.

Dairy Products

It has been said that we are the only species that never gets weaned. It is interesting to note, too, that cows' milk is quite different in composition from human milk. Even calves switch from udder to meadow in a short time. Many authorities are now calling into question our excessive use of milk, expecially the full-fat form, and its derivatives, including butter, cream, cheese, and ice cream. In addition, many adults are lactose intolerant, for them eating dairy products causes gastric disturbances.

Preservatives, Additives, Artificial Sweeteners, and Assorted Chemicals

Most of these products are not found in nature, but formulated in laboratories. Who can predict with certainty their long-range effect on our bodies? I don't want to be the guinea pig for this sort of experimentation. We all can cite instances of authorities labeling something as safe, only to change their minds in light of new research.

Salt

While sodium occurs naturally in many foods, there were no shakers from which to pour this contributor to hypertension and other health problems.

The Original Diet

What **did** our ancestors eat? Most experts agree that the primitive diet was primarily vegetarian, composed of what we now call complex carbohydrates. This family includes vegetables, tubers (comparable to today's white and sweet potatoes and yams), grains, roots, legumes (our beans, peas, and lentils), nuts, seeds, berries and other fruits. Animal flesh was eaten when the hunt was successful, when the salmon were running or other fish could be caught, or when a nest could be robbed of its eggs. Some honeycomb was probably added as a sweet treat when an individual was brave enough to get it.

What this program proposes is simply a return to this style of eating—the most health-supporting foods for our species. Advocacy of this high-complex carbohydrate, low-fat, low-cholesterol diet comes from no less prestigious source than the United States Select Committee on Nutrition and Human Needs. In addition, virtually every organization whose function it is to educate the public on the prevention of degenerative diseases share these views.

Experts may not agree on exact percentages. For the purposes of this plan, 60 to 80% of the food you eat should be complex carbohydrates, roughly 12% protein, and between 10 and 20% fats.

For further support, and regardless of one's religious beliefs, it is interesting to note that this healthiest of "diet plans" is precisely the one advocated in the Bible, Genesis 1:29: "I give you every seed-bearing plant on the face of the whole earth and every tree that has fruit with seed in it. They will be yours for food." The foods described are complex carbohydrates, whole and life-giving, perhaps because they themselves are alive.

The Benefits of Living Foods

Keep a carrot too long in the refrigerator, or forget a potato in the back of the cupboard, and what happens? It will sprout and grow. Beans and grains are seeds of plants; fruits and nuts have seeds inside them, and are capable of growth. A great tree begins from a tiny apple seed, a tall stalk from a single kernel of corn.

These are all foods that contain a life force—foods of the earth. It stands to reason that they are more health-promoting for our bodies than the "products" of factories. Try and sprout a doughnut, or watch a T.V. dinner grow. Such foods may have a place in our modern lives, but most assuredly should not be the major portion of our diets. Instead, we should eat as naturally as possible, with raw foods playing an important role. Unadulterated, unprocessed foods are best, the way they are found in nature, without being processed into another form. Try to keep to a minimum food items that come in bottles, cans, or jars. Read the label, and remember if you can't pronounce it, don't eat it.

Complex Carbohydrates—

Your "Home Base" Foods

Complex carbohydrates are the body's energy source. Since these healthful foods will comprise 60 to 80% of the foods you eat, it is important that you know a lot about them. And what a lucky time we live in! Not just on the coasts, but all across the country, fresh fruits and vegetables are the hottest sellers in the markets these days. In many places throughout the country the number of items in the produce section has tripled. The United Fresh Fruit and Vegetable Association's Supply Guide of available produce recently added seventy-five new fruits and vegetable items—and anything new and different is eagerly accepted by a willing public.

I routinely take my clients on two field trips. One is to a specialty produce market, or to the local supermarket with the finest quality fruits and vegetables; the second is to a health food store. These explorations are very important to their reeducation and subsequent success.

I come away from these field trips with the feeling that the lack of knowledge of what "healthy" foods really are, and what to do with them is a major contributor to years of improper eating and resulting overweight. Maybe you just didn't *know* what you were supposed to eat, and maybe your parents or your family doctor didn't either. When you have solid information and understanding of how to select and prepare new healthier foods, you will find it much easier to make the necessary changes in your diet, enjoy the process, and finally forgive yourself for years of being overweight.

Of course, reading books on the subject is helpful and highly recommended, but don't hesitate to ask a well-informed salesperson any of the questions that probably will come up in your early exploration of whole foods.

Make friends with your produce manager! He'll help you become familiar with the more exotic items. Learn when each fruit or vegetable is in its prime season, how to tell when the proper stage of ripeness has been reached, and how to select the best of the variety. Find out when produce is delivered, so you can schedule your shopping on the days that everything is freshest. When it is known that you are a willing student and appreciate quality, you might just have the ripest melon or the freshest mushrooms brought to you "from the back."

Which Produce is Best?

For fruits and vegetables, there is an order of preference: Fresh is almost always the best choice, but use your judgment. If the fresh vegetable looks past its prime, opt for the next best choice, which is frozen (with no added salt, sugar, or sauce). Canned foods are the least desirable—even those packed in their own juices.

SAMPLE WHOLE FOODS CONTINUUM
(from best to least desirable)

whole orange, picked from tree
whole orange, brought to market under ideal conditions
fresh squeezed orange juice, consumed immediately
re-constituted frozen, or juice in carton
canned orange juice
orange juice drink, or orangeade
powdered orange drinks (which contain hardly any fruit)

A Closer Look at Complex Carbohydrates

Fruits

Fruits are among the most healthful foods you can eat. They are high in potassium, but contain little or no sodium or fat. They are rich in fiber, vitamins, and minerals, and are very low in calories. It's just a bonus that they taste so delicious.

We are blessed with a magnificent variety of fruits from all parts of the earth to delight us with their sweetness. Our natural affinity for them is apparent—everybody loves *some* fruits, and some people, like me, never met a fruit they didn't like!

If you sometimes feel like eating only fruit as your whole meal, indulge yourself. Many former dieters have limited their fruit consumption, and welcome this "permission" to freely enjoy a food that comprised a major part of humankind's original diet.

When you hesitate to spend what seems like a lot of money for a beautiful pineapple or a special melon (try a special variety like Cranshaw, Canary or Sharlyn for a real treat), think of what you are saving on meat purchases. People just accept the fact that a good steak or roast will cost quite a lot, but will balk at being "extravagant" at the produce stand. Give that outdated concept some new thought, and treat yourself to the best!

Of course there is a variation in the number of calories among fruits, but generally they have such high water content and pack so much nutrition per calorie that you really don't need to concern yourself too much. Yes, even bananas (about 100 calories for a medium one) should be included for their potassium, fiber, and ability to fill you up.

I'm going to offer you just a partial list of the multitude of fruits available in most parts of the country. If you see one here or in the market that is new to you, make an effort to familiarize yourself with its virtues. It may become one of your favorites. Years ago, my best friend Susan introduced me to mangos, one of the most delicious tastes nature has to offer, and I am indebted to her forever.

All varieties of apples, bananas, oranges, grapefruits, tangerines, tangelos, mandarines, all varieties of grapes, melons, pears, plums, berries, including strawberries, raspberries, blackberries, blueberries, etc., peaches, nectarines, cherries, figs, pineapples, mangos, papayas, persimmons, kiwis, cherimoyas, guavas, passion fruit, Asian pear.

Dried fruits (without sulfur) are nutritionally dense, but also calorically dense. They should be used sparingly, but one or two pieces can sometimes satisfy a sweet tooth, or give a needed boost of energy. They require no refrigeration, and have been a favorite of back-packers for years. Tucked away in a purse or pocket, they make an excellent "fail-safe" snack to take along if you're in doubt about being able to eat when you get hungry (like on trips or in long meetings).

There is a form of processed dried fruit on the market called "fruit leather." Look for brands that are all natural and have no extra sweeteners or preservatives. These snacks are relatively low in calories, and neatly packed for convenience.

Vegetables

Vegetables are the lowest in calories of the complex carbohydrates—extremely nutritious and quite filling. As with fruits, learn everything you can. Don't pass up any vegetables in the market because you aren't familiar with them. Ask questions. Do you eat it raw or cooked? How do you select the best of its kind? Don't limit yourself to the old dieters' standbys of carrot sticks and celery. There are so many more from which to choose.

In this age of health and diet consciousness, raw vegetables (or crudités) are a popular hors d'oevre at social functions. In your own home, take care of yourself by making sure every time you open the refrigerator door, there they are, washed, peeled, cut up and ready. Nobody I know will come home starving, and start to peel carrots. Instead, people grab anything that's **ready**. But if a tempting array of vegetables was the first thing you spotted, you probably would munch on them while deciding what else to eat.

Try two of my favorites—peeled broccoli stems and red bell peppers. Did you know that a red bell pepper is a ripe green bell pepper? They are usually more expensive, but are much sweeter and have many more times the vitamin A content. Jicama, familiar in the west, is worth hunting for wherever you live. Peeled and eaten raw, it is crunchy and wonderful tasting. Some other vegetables good to serve raw include radishes, fennel, cauliflower, cucumbers, and zucchini.

Salad combinations are limited only by your imagination and the availability of produce. Please say goodbye to iceberg lettuce because it is of little nutritional value. The rule of thumb is the darker the vegetable (or fruit) the higher its nutritive content. In leafy vegetables this means that you are better off selecting romaine and other darker lettuces, spinach, collards, kale, chard, beet greens, parsley, etc. Then add any or all raw vegetables that look appealing at the store. Toss with a bit of lemon juice, one of the many surprisingly good-tasting no-oil dressings, or a light olive oil and good vinegar dressing, depending on how many calories you want to spend.

Make your salad big! Use a bowl that's supposed to serve four people. You can't eat too much of these life-giving foods. You can also expand that salad and make it into an entire meal. For example, add cooked brown rice, sprouts, cooked sliced potatoes, a small amount of cooked fish or lean meat, shellfish, sardines, tuna, a few sesame seeds, or raw nuts.

Some vegetables require light cooking, but don't overcook any vegetable. They should be *al dente,* like good pasta, with the exception of starchy members of the family like potatoes, yams, and winter squashes. Green beans, snow peas, asparagus, broccoli florets and Brussels sprouts do well lightly steamed. Stir frying (in the smallest possible amount of vegetable oil) and microwaving are acceptable. A huge platter of steamed vegetables is to be considered a "free" food for you to enjoy at will. Everyone loves corn on the cob, and it's amazing how quickly you can get used to it without butter.

Vegetables with Something Extra

Cruciferous vegetables are a special classification that have been cited for their anti-cancer properties. The group includes cabbage, broccoli, Brussels sprouts, cauliflower, collards, kale, turnip greens and kohlrabi.

Vegetables containing beta-carotene might also help to prevent cancer. These vegetables, all having a deep yellow or green color, include dark green leafies, carrots, beets, broccoli, pumpkin, yams and sweet potatoes, kale, collards, asparagus, tomatoes, and corn. As with salad ingredients, always look for vegetables of a comparatively deep color.

Starchy Vegetables

The starchy vegetables are very filling, and should become a mainstay of your healthy, low-calorie eating. Potatoes are not fattening! When high-fat toppings and sauces are left off, they are high-nutrition, low-calorie bargains. One day, have two medium-size baked potatoes and a cup of broth or other hot drink for lunch, and see how full you feel. You will be getting substantial amounts of fiber, vitamins, and minerals, but the calories will be low (100 calories in a five ounce potato).

Yams and sweet potatoes are a bit higher in calories, but delicious, filling, and very nutritious. They are excellent served hot, or eaten cold the next day. The winter squash (acorn, butternut, banana, spaghetti-squash and others) should also be on your menu, and can be seasoned with an assortment of herbs and spices instead of fat.

All potatoes and squash can be cooked basically the same way: bake them in about a 400 degree oven until soft when pierced with a fork. Or you can steam them, or follow microwave directions. Try baking other vegetables in a hot oven, without the addition of any sauce or fat. Chunks of carrots, eggplant, and Brussels sprouts are a few that are good this way. A whole unpeeled yellow onion baked until it is soft, loses its sharpness, and tastes very sweet.

An avocado is technically a fruit, but is most often eaten as a vegetable. Although it contains a number of vitamins and minerals, it is also high in fat and calories (1 cup of purée = 384 calories). If you want to include it in your diet, use very small quantities to give the desired flavor and richness. Try a tablespoonful as a topping for baked potatoes, or thinly spread on whole grain bread instead of mayonnaise (1 cup of mayonnaise = 1600 calories, so you're way ahead). Try a slice or two along side cold seafood, instead of a richer dressing.

Grains

This broad category includes breads, crackers, cereals, pasta, flour, corn, rice, barley, millet, buckwheat (kasha), oats, rye, wheat, popcorn, triticale (a high-protein cross between wheat and rye) and amaranth and quinoa, two highly nutritious ancient grains that have recently been "rediscovered."

These foods form the bulk of the diet of a large percentage of the world's population. Seek out these grain foods in their whole form, not bleached, refined, or instant.

Breads, Crackers, and Tortillas

Try to find whole grain foods made without shortening, oil, sugar or preservatives, although a small amount of a fat or sweetener in a whole grain product is acceptable. Be wary of crackers made with coconut or palm oil, which are saturated fats, and should be avoided.

Look for breads that say "100% whole grain flour" on the label. "100% wheat flour" can be all white flour with the valuable germ and bran removed, and is not the same as "100% whole wheat."

I urge you to move away from choosing plain white bread on a regular basis. When you eat whole grain breads, you get the nutritional benefits of the original grain, instead of a product stripped of many valuable nutrients and fiber. You can find some brands on the market that resemble the coarse, homemade loaves of earlier days. Or, you might bake your own whole grain bread, and enjoy the delicious aroma that fills your kitchen.

Cereals

There is a wide variety of hot and cold cereals available today containing the whole grain, but no fat, sugar, salt, or preservatives. They are wonderful for breakfast, and equally useful throughout the day.

Pasta

Pasta is one of the world's favorite foods, appearing in more shapes and forms than can be counted. The best is made from durum wheat, refined into flour called semolina. There are whole-grain "health" pastas on the market, but somehow, for me, they fall short of that true pasta taste. In this case I'd rather enjoy the real thing!

Coaches used to urge athletes to eat steak before a big game. Now the food of choice is often a large dish of energy-giving pasta. One cup of cooked pasta contains about 220 calories. With a no-oil sauce you can enjoy a true non-diet, delicious food.

Flours and Meals

This category includes whole wheat flour, whole wheat pastry flour, corn meal, buckwheat flour, and rye flour. Avoid white flour that has been stripped of virtually all its nutrients. "Enriching" means some nutrients are put back in during processing but why not get all the value of the original grain?

Whole Grains

Rice is a staple food for much of the world. But do limit your intake of white rice that has been stripped of most of its nutrients. Brown rice is more distinctive and richer tasting. Try long grain, medium or short grain brown rice, or the variations such as brown basmati rice or Wehani (with an extra dark, rich color and flavor). I know that Oriental restaurants serve white rice; enjoy it at those places, but cook with greater nutrient value in mind when you are at home.

Barley is excellent in soups and as a side dish. Rye is also very tasty when cooked like rice. Millet, buckwheat and triticale are exellent additions to your repertory.

Oats have always been a favorite breakfast cereal. They are also the principle ingredient of most granolas, but be careful, these blends can be higher in calories than commercial cereals because of the addition of sweeteners, nuts, dried fruits, and palm and coconut oil. You can make your own crunchy granola at home, and be in control of the ingredients.

Oat bran has been shown to have cholesterol-reducing properties because of its high content of water-soluble fiber. It was popularized as a hot cereal, but now also can be found in a dry crispy form, which many people prefer.

Corn in all its forms is a national favorite. Whether on the cob, frozen, as tortillas or corn meal, corn bread or corn muffins, keep the quantities of oil and butter down, and you have a family of nutritious and filling foods that can play a big part in your baseline diet.

Legumes

This broad group, including beans, peas, and lentils is an important component of the diet in many cultures. They are high protein, high fiber foods, but do not carry the fat baggage of other protein sources such as meat and cheese. They are amazingly versatile, very inexpensive, and can be stored indefinitely without refrigeration. Legumes contain high amounts of B vitamins and iron, two areas of deficiency in many American diets.

Some people are intimidated at the thought of cooking beans. While it is true that some do require a few hours to reach the desired stage of softness, the cook is not actively involved. Once they are picked over, rinsed, covered with water and set on the stove, they take care of themselves. I have never found the need to pre-soak beans before cooking, but please check some of the many comprehensive vegetarian or health-oriented cookbooks to learn the few simple techniques necessary to incorporate these valuable foods into your diet.

Lentils are exceptions to the long cooking requirement. They can be ready in well under thirty minutes, making a hearty soup or stew, depending on how much water you add.

Soy beans, the backbone of many Asian cuisines, are

amazingly versatile. They are the source of textured vegetable protein, used commercially in many products; tofu, the white soy bean curd that comes in a little square and its taste varies according to its use; soy oil; and even ice cream-like desserts, such as Toffutti. Read the labels carefully on those products. Some of them have as many calories and as much fat as regular ice cream. They are healthier only in that they are of plant origin and contain no cholesterol.

Since you will be limiting your use of meats, it's important to get to know and like many different kinds of legumes. They can create satisfying and delicious dishes that seem to warm the heart as well as the stomach. Think of minestrone or split pea soup, baked beans, Mexican-style pintos, lima bean casserole, black beans and rice. All of these and more can be cooked in a non-fat or low-fat way, and still taste wonderful. Some of the other varieties you might try are navy, mung, kidney, great northern, and adzuki beans, garbanzos (chick peas), and black-eyed peas.

Sprouts

The sprouts of grains, seeds and legumes are miniature powerhouses of nutrition. When a seed sprouts, the germination causes an enormous increase in the already high nutritional value across the board—vitamins, minerals, and protein. The sprouting process also makes them more digestible, and their nutrients easier for the body to absorb. There are probably even more health benefits as yet undiscovered, because these foods are truly filled with life.

Sprouts are low in calories, high in fiber, and very inexpensive to buy. Many markets here in California stock them as a staple of the produce department. But growing them youself is easy, and assures you a constant supply at just the right stage of development. Children love to help in this project, because results are visible in twenty-four hours, and the "harvest" is ready in a couple of days at most. It is a fun way to introduce them to natural foods.

Almost any kind of legume, seed or grain will sprout successfully, with very little special equipment or care. Instructions telling you how to get started can be found in many natural food books, and the simple equipment you need will be in your health food store. The basic procedure is to soak the grain or legume for a few hours, then drain the water (use it to water your house plants!), then rinse the sprouts three times a day.

Some popular varieties you can try include wheat, rye, mung bean, adzuki bean, lentil, garbanzo, sunflower, and black-eyed peas.

Add them to salads, or nibble them as a between meal snack. Sprouted grains are excellent in morning cereal. I especially like sprouted rye or wheat as part of my breakfast, and add sprouted lentils and other legumes to almost every salad.

Nuts and Seeds

These delicious nuggets are notoriously easy to eat. A cup of peanuts or cashews can be gone before you know it. Although they are rich sources of vegetable protein and contain valuable nutrients and healthy kinds of fats, their calorie count is quite high. Therefore they must be used in moderation. No more handfuls at cocktail time! (Try air-popped popcorn instead.) But a few nuts judiciously sprinkled on the low-calorie vegetable portions of a meal can add a lot of flavor. Some examples: a few cashews on a Chinese-type stir-fry or chicken salad; almonds used sparingly to top breakfast cereal or yogurt; sesame seeds sprinked over a rice dish.

It is much healthier to eat all nuts and seeds in their raw state, not roasted or salted. Peanuts, not truly nuts, but legumes, should always be roasted before eating.

A brief list of nuts and seeds includes: walnuts, pistachios, almonds, cashews, pignolas (pine nuts), pecans, macademias, brazils, filberts (also called hazelnuts), sesame, pumpkin, caraway, poppy, sunflower, and flax seeds.

A glance at their caloric content should keep you prudent in the use of this food group:

½ cup chopped walnuts	391 calories
4 oz. hulled pumpkin seeds	627 calories
4 shelled brazil nuts	114 calories

Fiber

Mothers and grandmothers used to tell us to eat "rough-age." Once again, as is so often the case, yesterday's folk wisdom is todays scientific recommendation. Today most experts are urging us to increase our intake of foods containing abundant roughage, now called by its new name—fiber.

No animal products contain fiber. These foods are totally digested and absorbed into the body as calories. Fiber can only be found in plant foods—yet another reason for following a high complex-carbohydrate diet.

Fiber serves an important purpose in controlling weight. When you eat high-fiber foods, you get fuller, faster. Three ounces of steak, a very small portion costs you 300 calories. After the few bites it takes to finish the serving, you're left wondering what else to eat. For the same number of calories, you can "buy" a five-ounce baked potato, practically unlimited quantities of salad (with a no-oil dressing), a cup of steamed broccoli, and an apple. While that might not be your meal of choice, there is no question that after eating it, you will feel full. Put very simply, eating foods higher in fiber allows you the pleasure of eating more quantity.

Diets that prescribe half-portions of high-fat, low-fiber foods must fail in the long run. No one will tolerate feeling half-hungry most of the time. Your diet will be over as soon as your will power breaks down. It is much more sensible and kind to yourself to make it your goal never to feel empty and deprived. Instead, fill up on low-calorie, high-bulk foods.

In addition to the filling value of fiber-rich foods, they are also recommended by doctors for the prevention of a long list of ailments, including constipation, hemorrhoids, and diver-ticulosis. A diet rich in fiber, particularly wheat bran, tends to normalize the action of the intestines by moving food rapidly through the digestive tract. Everyone feels better when elimina-tion is functioning smoothly.

Increasingly, diabetics, ulcer sufferers, and patients with heart disease are also urged to increase their consumption of high-fiber foods.

Oat bran, and other foods with water-soluble fiber have been shown to be effective in reducing cholesterol levels. Additional sources of this beneficial type of fiber include black-eyed peas and other beans, peas, corn, sweet potatoes and pears.

Simple carbohydrates, including baked goods derived from white flour, sugars, and candy, have been stripped of their fiber as well as most of their nutrients. It is in the family of *complex carbohydrates* that we find this vital dietary component.

Heading the list of rich sources of fiber are the grains, including wheat, oats, rice, barley, corn, millet, and the products made from them. Unprocessed wheat bran has the most fiber of all. It can be sprinkled on cereals and salads, mixed into yogurt, or added to casseroles or other prepared foods. Start with one or two tablespoons to see how your system reacts to the increased fiber intake.

Legumes, nuts, seeds, vegetables and fruits also contain fiber. Since root vegetables, especially potatoes are so filling, whole meals can be built around them.

The correlation is clear: the fewer no-fiber foods you eat (meat, eggs, cheese, oil, butter, cakes, candies, pastries), and the more high-fiber foods that are in your diet (brown rice, whole wheat products, potatoes, vegetables, fruits, and salads), the more likely you are to enjoy an ideal, stable body weight, along with measurably improved health.

Other Components of Our Food

Protein

If the average American were stopped on the street and asked "What is the most important type of food for you to eat?" the answer would most likely be protein. Most of us have been convinced through the years that protein should be predominant over other dietary components, and that the "best" protein comes from animal sources. So we dutifully consume large quantities of meats, milk, eggs, and cheese. While it is quite true that these foods are high in protein, they carry with them the heavy baggage of fat, cholesterol, and a lot of calories.

Protein is made up of amino acids, which can be found both in animal products and in foods that come from plants. By including in your diet a wide variety of grains, fruits, vegetables, and legumes, you will have absolutely no problem getting a sufficient quantity of these necessary amino acids. In fact, while getting adequate protein is essential for good health, the Center for Science in the Public Interest in Washington says that the actual consumption of total protein in the U.S. is about double what we need. It appears that as long as we get enough calories, we need not worry about getting enough protein. Many people are surprised when they learn that "energy"—the body's actual fuel—comes not from protein, but from carbohydrates.

Consuming no animal protein at all is a viable eating style practiced by large populations of the world. To too many people, however, it remains a startling thought that the evening meal does not need a slab of meat as its focal point. The fact is that foods long considered side dishes can stand on their own as delicious, satisfying meals.

Animal protein, when and if you choose to have it, should be thought of as a condiment, rather than the meal's centerpiece. The portion that you once served one person can now serve the entire family, or can be cut, wrapped and frozen for future use.

Oriental cultures approach animal protein foods in a healthier fashion than we do. In a Chinese restaurant, most dishes start with lots of crisp-tender vegetables and rice, then small quantities of meat or fish may be added.

When I was a child, I went to the butcher shop with my mother. Prominently displayed on the wall above the meat case was a sign that read "A meal without meat is a meal incomplete." A catchy phrase to be sure, but a concept that is out of favor with people interested in good health. Support for this point of view comes from reliable data showing that Seventh Day Adventists, most of whom eat no meat or poultry, have substantially lower incidents of heart disease and cancer.

When you do choose to serve beef, veal, or lamb, eat small portions of the leanest cuts. Fish, chicken, and turkey are generally lower in fat, but should also be eaten in small quantities, and not necessarily every day.

Fish
Fish is coming into favor as the superior choice among animal proteins. The fat it contains is the polyunsaturated kind,

and some species have been shown to contain omega-3 fatty acids, a substance that may protect against heart disease. While the waters of our planet have been polluted in varying degrees, they appear to be a better overall risk as a food source than the feed lots and confined cages of bred-for-food animals, where hormone, steroid, and antibiotic innoculations are routine.

Our waters contain enormous varieties of fish and other seafood. Rapid transportation and modern freezing techniques make many choices available year 'round. If your idea of a fish dinner has thus far been frozen fish sticks, explore some new possibilities. Most people like shellfish, especially shrimp, lobster and crab, but these foods have the drawbacks of being somewhat high in cholesterol, and often prohibitively expensive. Swordfish, halibut, sea bass, shark, salmon, and many other firm-textured varieties have virtually no "fishy" taste or smell, are either boneless or easily filleted, and are good starting points for red-meat eaters learning to expand their horizons.

Fats

Most people still believe that sugar is the number one enemy when it comes to fighting overweight. In reality, fats of all kinds are two and one-fourth times more caloric than sugar and are the greater problem. Fats are calories packaged in their most concentrated form, containing nine calories per gram, while proteins and carbohydrates contain four calories per gram. High-fat diets almost invariably create fat bodies.

Diets rich in fat, especially the saturated kind found mostly in animal products, are implicated as risk factors for cardiovascular disease, diabetes, and some forms of cancer. With so many compelling reasons to decrease the fat in our diet, why do we eat so much of it?

The fact is that fats make food taste good. Many people's list of favorite foods include one high-fat entry after another: steak, cheese, ice cream, pie, pizza, and chocolate. A hostess who wants to be praised as a great cook has half the battle won with the liberal use of butter, oil, and cream. The main reason people patronize one eating place over another is simply because they think the food tastes better. Heavy uses of fats and sugar are the surest way to please the public taste and guarantee high profits—obviously the route chosen by the fast food industry.

Since fats contain no fiber at all, they "slip down" easily, taking up little room in the stomach. They don't offer much in the way of pleasure from the act of chewing and subsequent feelings of fullness, yet their caloric price is very high. Some examples of the "high cost" of fatty foods:

1 tbs. butter	100 calories
1 tbs. any oil	120 calories
1 cup shelled brazil nuts	916 calories
4 oz. Hershey Bar	623 calories

——————Some comparisons (approximate):

1 cup flour	450 calories
1 cup sugar	750 calories
1 cup butter	1600 calories
1 cup oil	2000 calories

——————some substitutions:

INSTEAD OF:	YOU COULD HAVE:	CALORIES
1 oz. (1 inch square) cheddar cheese	2 cups of strawberries	100
2 oz. pastrami	A 3 oz. Sealtest ice cream sandwich	170
1 cup cocktail peanuts	34 cups of air-popped popcorn	800

With this information in mind, it becomes essential to get rid of as much fat as possible in your menus. Some fats are necessary for good health, but they can be found in a variety of whole foods, including grains, legumes, nuts, seeds and avocados, without the addition of extra fats.

Where's the Fat?

Many fats are quite visible: the white part around the edge of meat and the marbeling running through it; the yellow chicken fat beneath the skin. Butter, most margarines, vegetable shortening, lard, and all oils are 100% fat. Many hard cheeses are up to 80% fat, and should not be considered as primarily protein foods. Sausages, bacon, mayonnaise, and whole milk are major sources of fat in the diet.

Most fats are shiny. Look for the tell-tale glistening on the bottom of salad bowls, including pasta and vegetable salads, in the broiler pan after cooking meats, on the surface of unskimmed soups and stews and wherever butter, margarine, or oil are used.

Other fats are hidden, as in rich "flaky" pastries, ice cream, chocolate, and nuts. Stay away from fried foods. They absorb large quantities of fat from the frying medium, multiplying their original calorie count. Some fast-food companies use beef fat to fry their potatoes and chicken, and those fats are used over and over again. Whan an unappetizing concept!

Become very aware of how much fat there is in common foods. Read labels. While only animal fats contain cholesterol, from the standpoint of calories, all types are about the same— saturates, polyunsaturates, and monounsaturates. Of all the popular oils, olive oil, a monounsaturate, is getting the best press these days because it may be effective in lowering total cholesterol while preserving the "good" (or HDL) cholesterol, thus reducing the risk of heart attack. The people of Greece and Southern Italy *do* have a lower rate of heart problems, and have known for years that olive oil is the tastiest of the oils. Its delicious flavor goes a long way, so even a teaspoonful can add a lot of enjoyment to a prepared food or a salad.

Sugar

While not as caloric as fats, be wary of another group of foods: the sugars—white and brown sugar, honey, molasses, maple syrup, turbinado and raw sugar. These are the simple sugars of simple carbohydrates that lack the high nutritional value of their complex counterparts. They are quickly absorbed by the body, and seem only to increase hunger; they especially increase your need for more sweets. Sweet foods are calorically dense. A little bit adds up to a lot of calories, but since you don't feel full, you tend to go on eating. A box of chocolates is very easy to polish off in one sitting.

Often, people who eat lots of sweets don't manage to get enough healthy foods in their diet—a condition described as being overfed and undernourished. Some theorists believe that it is the body's need for missing nutrients that perpetuates a continuous state of hunger, as though the indiscriminate foraging must go on until the right nutrients are supplied. But the predictable outcome of eating large quantities of the wrong foods is obesity, a prime risk-factor for many degenerative diseases.

Even if you never spoon sugar from a bowl, you still may be eating a lot more than you realize. Hidden sugars are in baked goods, candy, ice cream, soft drinks, and many other foods that may surprise you, such as ketchup and sauces. Read every label of every food that goes into your body and be alert for sugar in all its forms. Some words indicating sugar content are: fructose, maltose, lactose, glucose, dextrose, and corn syrup.

One twelve-ounce soft-drink contains six to nine teaspoons of sugar, while a small piece of chocolate layer cake has up to fifteen teaspoons. That's a lot of empty calories working hard to add fat to your body but making no contribution to your health and vitality. Here's some good news: many people report that after eating a healthy, more natural diet, the sweet cravings that used to haunt them either go away or are greatly diminished.

Salt

By now, everyone is aware that too much salt in the diet is not healthy. Sodium (table salt is a combination of sodium and chloride) is implicated as a major contributor to hypertension, more commonly called high blood pressure.

The body does require some sodium, but only a tiny fraction of what the average American diet provides. This need is easily met by eating a diet high in natural foods, with nothing additional from the shaker.

Even if you are careful about adding salt to your food, you still may be consuming too much. The latest American Heart Association recommendation is that we cut sodium intake to less than one level teaspoon a day. This may be difficult since salt is the most popular additive, used in quantity in fast foods and in almost every processed food. Chips, cocktail nuts, pretzels, pickles, and anchovies are obvious sources, but it also turns up in surprising places like canned soups, frozen dinners, and even boxes of cereal (another reason to read every label).

Excess salt and rich foods seem to go hand in hand. Changing to a diet emphasizing more natural foods is one way to eliminate the problem. "Purer" foods seem better able to stand on their own, especially with the addition of spices, herbs, lemon juice, vinegar, mustard, or salsa used as salt substitutes.

Since the taste for salty foods is an acquired one, it can be modified over time. After following a more natural diet for a while, some commercially salted foods taste truly inedible. I tried some salted mixed nuts at a party recently, and thought there must have been some mistake. I felt like I was eating salt by the spoonful.

Some people use this additive so unthinkingly that they automatically salt their food before tasting it. While you are in the process of changing your tastes, never add salt to food while cooking. Wait until it is served, taste it, and then if you must, salt the surface.

Excess sodium intake can cause fluid retention, and a consequent "false" weight gain. If you indulge in a high-sodium meal—a fast-food chicken dinner or a pizza with pepperoni, you could wake up the next morning with an increased scale weight of three to four pounds! This is a gain of water, not fat. There are 3,500 calories in a pound of fat, and it is unlikely that you consumed 14,000 calories the day before.

This sort of bizarre scale reading is one reason why I am against daily weigh-ins. Seeing such an increase on the scale the "morning after" could have dangerous consequences for someone who didn't understand the difference between retaining fluid and adding fat. You could come to the conclusion that the minute you "break your diet," and eat any foods simply for fun you get fat anyway so you might as well give up the struggle.

I certainly am not advocating high-sodium consumption, but barring any medical problems, this sort of episode can be balanced over time into your long-range eating plan, and need not be the cause of depression and feelings of failure.

How Your Tastes Will Change

An Eskimo child regards blubber as a treat, while a young Bantu searches under a log for the insects he considers a delicacy. Neither choice appeals to us, yet these people inhabit the same earth as we do, and possess identical digestive equipment. It becomes obvious that while we all share the biological hunger drive, custom and habit play an overwhelming part in what we eat, and habits can be changed.

Susie, an aspiring young actress, predicted it would be impossible to kick her addiction to French fries. A few months later however, she reported that they were no longer tempting to her, and wondered why she wasted so many calories on them over the years.

Barbara, a public relations executive and former "carnivore," ate a large steak at a business lunch after not having red meat for many months. She said she felt "heavy" and distressed after the meal, describing herself as a python who had devoured a whole animal and had a protruding hump in the middle of its body.

Just by following a more natural diet, modifications in your tastes will occur spontaneously. Some foods will seem rich, greasy, or overly sweet, leading you to wonder whether somebody changed the recipes of former favorites. Actually, it will be you who did the changing. Taste buds are distorted by a steady diet of fats, sugar, and chemicals. When those substances play a smaller part in your diet, purer, more natural flavors come through, and the old foods taste "foreign." In fact, some people report that the aromas coming from fast food places were once a tantalizing invitation for some serious eating, but now, all they smell is reused fat, and it totally turns them off.

Although fried foods and red meat are the foods that most frequently lose their appeal over time, the love of certain foods never dies; you will just crave them with decreasing frequency. I read a quote attributed to John Denver: "I have ice cream any time I feel like it. I just feel like it less and less."

One of my more memorable patients was a comedy writer named Marty. When I first saw him, he weighed 360 pounds, and was under strict medical supervision. My job was to teach him an entirely new approach to food.

Of course he had been eating large quantities of fatty foods. (It is difficult to get to 360 pounds without them.) Fast foods and fried foods, doughnuts and cheese were his major sustenance. The world of complex carbohydrates was completely new, and the reeducation process took many months.

One day, I knew we were both on the road to success. Marty had bought himself an inexpensive stainless steel steamer, and was experimenting with a variety of vegetables. Very seriously, with none of his usual humor, he informed our nutrition class that crisp tender broccoli was the best, carrots were delicious, and that beets turned the steaming water bright red.

The most significant revelation was that all afternoon while at work, Marty found himself looking forward to having the vegetables and the brown rice that would accompany them. That night he wanted that particular meal more than a cheeseburger. No longer was he depriving himself of what he really wanted and eating only what he "should." His own "organic" choices had changed.

In no way does this imply that Marty will never again want his former staples, nor that he will never have them, but the best predictor of success in lifetime weight management is that moment when the realization dawns that you like, and indeed sometimes prefer, the foods that are good for you an increasing percentage of the time.

Tastes are modified in an evolutionary way. Think of what you used to eat as a child. Perhaps the recollections of some foods or meals are surrounded by warm memories or unpleasant ones, but either way, it is unlikely that you are regularly eating many of those same foods today.

Next year's foods will probably be somewhat different from what you eat right now. New products come on the market, we learn more about nutrition, your body has different needs. Pick up the reins of control. Modify your eating habits to conform to your desire for a slim body and a high level of health, and be confident that it is only a matter of time before these foods become exactly what you want to eat most of the time.

References

Bailey, Covert.
    1977. *Fit or Fat?* Boston: Houghton Mifflin Co.
    1989. *The Fit or Fat Woman.* Boston: Houghton Mifflin Co.
Ballentine, Rudolph.
    1978. *Diet and Nutrition.* Honesdale, PA: Himalayan International Institute.
Barnett, Robert.
    1986. "Why Fat Makes You Fatter." *American Health Magazine*, (May, 1986): 38–41.
Brody, Jane E.
    1981. *Jane Brody's Nutrition Book.* New York: W.W. Norton.
    1985. *Jane Brody's Good Food Book.* New York: W.W. Norton.
    1986. "Fitness: Is It Good For You?" *The Good Health Magazine*, *N.Y. Times*, (September 28): 24–99.
Carroll, David.
    1985. *The Complete Book of Natural Foods.* New York: Summit Books.
Danforth, E.
    1985. "Diet and Obesity." *American Journal of Clinical Nutrition*, 41:1132–1145.
Eaton, S. Boyd, Marjorie Shostak and Melvin Konner.
    1988. *The Paleolithic Prescription.* New York: Harper & Row.
Elliot, Rose.
    1988. *Complete Vegetarian Cuisine.* New York: Random House.
Flatt, J. P.
    1987. "Dietary Fat, Carbohydrate Balance, and Weight Maintenance; Effects of Exercise." *American Journal of Clinical Nutrition*, 45:296–306.
Fonda, Jane.
    1984. *Women Coming of Age.* New York: Simon & Schuster.
Goldstein, Sue.
    1987. *The Underground Shopper's Guide to Health and Fitness.* New York: Fawcett Columbine.
Greenwald, Jerry.
    1974. *Be The Person You Were Meant To Be.* New York: Simon & Schuster.
Haigh, Rachel.
    1987. *The Neal's Yark Bakery Whole Food Cookbook.* Topsfield, MA: Salem House.
Kenton, Leslie and Susannah.
    1984. *Raw Energy.* New York: Warner Books.
Kowalski, Robert.
    1987. *The 8 Week Cholesterol Cure.* New York: Harper & Row.
Lawrence, D. H.
    1911. *The White Peacock.* New York: Viking (Cambridge Edition Texts: 1985).
Liebman, Bonnie.
    1989. "Calories Don't Count Equally." *Nutrition Action Health Letter*, (Jan/Feb., 1989): 8–9.
Long, Patricia J. and Barbara Shannon.
    1983. *Nutrition, An Inquiry Into The Issues.* Englewood Cliffs, N.J.: Prentice Hall.

MacNeil, Karen.
 1981. *The Book of Whole Foods, Nutrition and Cuisine*. New
   York: Vintage Books.
Mayer, Jean and Jeanne Goldberg.
 1987. "University Studies Show Body Size Is All In The Family." Los Angeles Times, (Oct. 15, 1987): 31.
McDougall, John.
 1983. *The McDougall Plan*. Piscataway, N.J.: New Century
   Publishers.
Meer, Jeff.
 1986. "Breaking With Breakfast." *Psychology Today*, (August): 6.
Mirkin, Gabe.
 1983. *Getting Thin*. Boston: Little, Brown & Co.
———.
 1981. National Institute of Health Study. Reported in *Journal of
   the American Medical Association*, (Jan. 23/30:1981):
   371–373.
Pauling, Linus.
 1970. *Vitamin C and the Common Cold*. San Francisco: W. H.
   Freeman.
Perls, Frederick, Ralph F. Hefferline and Paul Goodman.
 1977. *Gestalt Therapy*. New York: Bantam Books.
Piscatella, Joseph.
 1987. *Choices for A Healthy Heart*. New York: Workman.
Remington, Dennis W., Garth A. Fisher and Edward Parent.
 1983. *How To Lower Your Fat Thermostat*. Provo, UT: Vitality
   House International.
Robbins, John.
 1987. *Diet For a New America*. Walpole, NH: Stillpoint.
Robertson, Laurel, Carol Flinders and Bronwen Godfrey.
 1976. *Laurel's Kitchen*. Berkeley: Nilgiri Press.
Saltman, Paul, Joel Gurin and Ira Mothner.
 1987. The California Nutrition Book. Boston: Little, Brown & Co.
Sims, E. A. H.
 1986. "Energy Balance in Human Beings: The Problem of Plen-
   titude." *Vitamins & Hormones*, Vol. 43. San Diego/Or-
   lando/New York: Academic Press.
———.
   Tufts University Diet and Nutrition Newsletter. Published
   monthly. 55 Park Place, N.Y., N. Y. 10007.
———.
 1985. University of Kansas Study (Research by Lisa I. McCann
   and David S. Holmes) cited in *Vegetarian Times Magazine*, (May, 1985): 17.
———.
   University of California, Berkeley Wellness Letter. Published Monthly. P.O. Box 359162, Palm Coast, Florida.
Ward, Alex.
 1984. "Athletes: Older But Fitter," *N.Y. Times Magazine*, (Oct.
   28, 1984): 90–98.
Whitaker, Julian.
 1985. *Reversing Heart Disease*. New York: Warner.
 1987. *Reversing Diabetes*. New York: Warner.